Building Health
by DESIGN

To Constance,

May you optimize your health
+ maximize your life!

Building Health
by DESIGN

Adding Life to Your Years
and Years to Your Life!

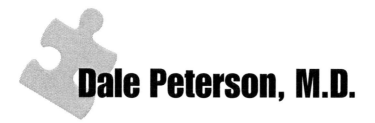

Dale Peterson, M.D.

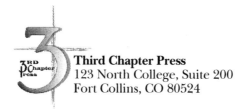

Third Chapter Press
123 North College, Suite 200
Fort Collins, CO 80524

Copyright © 2010 by Dale Peterson, M.D.
Health by Design
1006 West Taft, #342
Sapulpa, OK 74066
email: info@drdalepeterson.com
Website: www.drdalepeterson.com

ISBN-13: 978-0-9830129-4-8
ISBN-10: 0-9830129-4-6

Printed in the United States of America

All Scripture quotations, unless otherwise indicated, are taken from the *New King James Version*. Copyright © 1982 by Thomas Nelson, Inc. Used by permission. All rights reserved.

Cover Designer & Typesetter: Michelle Kenny, Fort Collins, CO

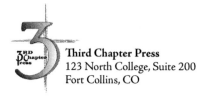
Third Chapter Press
123 North College, Suite 200
Fort Collins, CO

Dedication

*This book is dedicated to my mother, Phyllis Peterson,
without whose encouragement I would not have attended
college and pursued a career in medicine.*

Table of Contents

Foreword

Dr. Dale Peterson is one of the best informed and most knowledgeable medical practitioners in America today. His initial impact was made in the mainline medical community as a professor at the University of Wisconsin and University of Oklahoma Colleges of Medicine, President of the Oklahoma Academy of Family Physicians, and in his own private medical clinic. His impact now continues in the lives and wellbeing of those who are wise enough to read this book.

His insight into the cause and proliferation of human illnesses led him to look beyond standard medical practice into research pathways where he could anticipate cures, rather than routinely treat patient symptoms. His knowledge of the profound interrelationship between the physical body and the inner health of the individual led him to discover, and appropriate, positive patient results a full league beyond standard medical practice or alternative medical procedures.

This book characterizes and details myriad problems with our current medical practices that encourage unconscionable suffering in our "enlightened" society. As Dr. Peterson observes, "We don't have an active disease prevention system in this country; we have a disease promotion system." In *Building Health by Design* he explains why diseases that are common in our society rarely develop when the body's intrinsic healing mechanisms are properly supported.

In this volume, among other things, the reader is made aware of the benefits of *pure energized water* and its role in the health of the individual. The detrimental significance of free radicals is discussed, encouraging a life-changing awareness. The amazing benefits of enzymes are explored and emphasized. To the surprise of many, insightful explanation is given to show that "acute inflammation can promote healing; chronic inflammation can lead to a wide range of disease states and a significant acceleration of the aging process."

Dr. Peterson discovered that the human body is actually designed to heal itself. This beautiful symphony of the human personality and the Creator's provision embodies a response in the human spirit reminiscent of being in partnership with the Creator Himself. In fact, this insightful book will detail the steps by which you can routinely live in concert with the Designer of the human body and the unique purpose He has outlined for your life and wellbeing.

Dr. Peterson doesn't attempt to overwhelm the reader with his vast knowledge of the medical literature and his familiarity with technical descriptions; he graciously sits at your kitchen table as a compassionate Christian physician who has come to your home with your personal wellbeing at heart. He is about "wellness."

This timely volume should be required reading in every college curriculum and hold a place of preferred reference in every Christian home. The author shows the reader how to "treat your body like a palace—not a garbage dump." With the diagnosis and practices described in these pages, he actually saved his own life. Now, with the application of the information offered herein, this book can save your life!

—Carl E. Baugh, Ph.D., Founder and Director,
Creation Evidence Museum, Glen Rose, Texas

Preface

*I will praise You, for I am fearfully and **wonderfully** made; Marvelous are Your works, And that my soul knows very well.*
– Psalm 139:14

"I am fearfully and wonderfully made." It has been three thousand years since those words were originally written, but the truth they express is more evident today than ever. I appreciate their meaning more with each passing day.

I have been studying the design of the human body for over forty years. I use the word "design" intentionally, for the human body could not have evolved by chance. It is structural, having tissues and organs. It is biochemical, with a nearly infinite number of reactions occurring at any point in time. It is electrical; life is defined by the presence of electrical activity in the heart and brain. The body is magnetic, relying on the earth's electromagnetic field as its primary energy source.

We human beings are more than bodies, however. Each of us has a soul and a spirit. The soul, comprised of the mind, will, and emotions, gives each person a unique personality. The spirit gives life to the body. David was correct in his assessment of the human condition—each of us is fearfully and wonderfully made.

Scientific medicine rejects the concept that the human body was carefully and marvelously designed by a wise and benevolent Creator. Evolutionary theory was the basis of my formal education from elementary school through medical school. It remains at the core of the continuing medical education courses I take each year.

Evolutionary theory is not capable of providing answers to common health challenges. It takes a fatalist approach to the challenge of disease and aging. Disease, it seems, just happens; it is the unfortunate result of flaws within the body, of having been dealt a poor genetic hand in the game of life. Evolutionary medicine states that the reason my father died of a heart attack was that his body contained too much "bad cholesterol"—he had not evolved from his hunter-gatherer past quickly enough to survive in an industrial/informational society.

Building health by design takes an optimistic approach to disease and aging. Disease doesn't "just happen"; it is the result of specific challenges to the body's integrity that can be successfully countered by supporting the body's intrinsic, God-given healing mechanisms. The design approach to disease states that the reason my father died from a heart attack was that his body was not given the raw materials required to respond to inflammation in his arteries and to prevent oxidative damage to his LDL cholesterol.

Approximately twenty-five years ago, I made the decision to approach the challenge of disease from a viewpoint of design rather than from the standard evolutionary position. The results have been beyond anything I could have imagined at the time. Today I routinely see what I would have considered miracles in my former way of approaching illness. They are miracles, but they are miracles not of a suspension of the laws of nature, but of the incredible healing mechanisms that are part of the body's design.

This is a book about the design of the human body, the mechanisms that lead to disease and accelerate aging, and how supporting the intrinsic, God-given healing mechanisms within the body can restore and maintain vitality and add years to one's life.

Acknowledgements

I thank my wife, Rosalie, along with my children and grandchildren who have stood by me while I have taken a road less travelled. Without their love and support I could not have persevered. I am grateful to the many fellow travelers on the road to wellness who have consulted me over the years, challenging me to continually seek additional ways to restore and maintain health. I thank Dr. Carl Baugh for challenging my world view and encouraging me to integrate my belief in a Creator into my approach to healing. I am indebted to Brian Klemmer and his associates for facilitating the renewing of my mind. I appreciate Fred Van Liew's ongoing study of energetic protective appliances and thank him for introducing me to the concept of checking the body's central computer. I am grateful to Doris Stearman for her assistance in framing technical material in a manner that can be grasped by readers without a scientific background. Most of all I thank קדש את־רוח who has been my constant Companion, Instructor, and Guide in my quest to understand the design of the human body, the mechanisms of disease and aging, and the steps that can be taken to address them.

Chapter 1
The Importance of Keeping an Open Mind

Enter by the narrow gate; for wide is the gate and broad is the way that leads to destruction, and there are many who go in by it. Because narrow is the gate and difficult is the way which leads to life, and there are few who find it.
– Matthew 7:13-14

My Worldview

I believe the Judeo-Christian Bible records the inspired and infallible words of the living God. My belief in the Creator who designed the human body in His likeness and my desire to please Him govern all aspects of my life, including my approach to the health challenges for which people come to me for assistance.

I make my worldview known at the outset, because I believe how one looks at life makes a difference. I also state it because, ironically, Bible-believing Christians, who profess a belief in God, are among those least willing to embrace healing by design. I am frequently asked, "If you are really a Christian how can you practice alternative medicine?" as though the two are incompatible. I explain that I don't practice alternative medicine, but rather offer people alternatives to medicine. I know, however, that misses the point of the question. I know that most Christians are very close-minded when exposed to concepts that sound or look strange to them. While not explicitly expressed, they believe energy points to be inexorably linked to Eastern mysticism. To speak of chakras, meridians, and the body's innate intelligence is to operate in the realm of the occult—to heal, as Jesus was accused of doing, by the power of Beelzebub.

Open or Close-mindedness; Narrow or Broad-mindedness

We filter new ideas and information as they are presented to us. The four major filters are open-mindedness, close-mindedness, narrow-mindedness, and broad-mindedness. If you are open-minded, you will be willing to consider the possibility that the idea has merit. You are willing to study the subject further, even if it means that you will need to make changes in your life. If you are close-minded, you will reject new concepts out-of-hand if they do not line up with your current way of looking at things.

If you are narrow-minded, you believe that truth exists and that there are moral absolutes. If you are narrow-minded, you will further filter the new information through the light of the fundamental principles that guide your approach to life. If the concept violates those principles, it will be rejected. If, on the other hand, you are broad-minded, you believe that absolute truth does not exist and that moral values are relative. If you are broad-minded, you will not question the validity of the information in light of any fundamental truth.

I encourage my Christian readers to keep an open mind. When Jesus taught that His followers should enter by the narrow gate, He was not telling them to be close-minded. He was telling them to be narrow-minded, which is something quite different. As a follower of Jesus, I am challenged to be very open-minded, to be willing to look at anything that might provide more insight into how to help others. I am, however, to be narrow-minded, weighing concepts that are new to me in the light of His word. The result is personal growth and a greater appreciation of His creative ability.

Why Physicians Are Reluctant to Embrace the Concept of Building Health by Design

Christians are not the only people who tend to be close-minded when it comes to building health by design. Physicians are among the most close-minded people in the world. As I speak to groups across the country, I am frequently asked, "Why aren't more doctors recommending non-pharmacologic or non-surgical approaches to health problems?" While there are undoubtedly many factors involved, I believe that lack of knowledge is by far the most significant.

Nearly every individual who enters medical school does so because of a desire to heal and be of service to others. When physicians recommend drugs, surgery, radiation, or other treatment options, they are, with rare exception, doing so because they believe that they are acting in the best interest of the individual seeking their assistance. The failure to approach problems in a manner that supports the body's ability to heal rather than in a manner that is injurious to the body is not due to a lack of compassion. It is due to a system of undergraduate, post-doctoral, and continuing medical education that at best ignores and at worst ridicules the use of nutritional and energetic measures to restore and maintain health.

It is difficult for a traditional Christian who has been taught that any method of healing that emerged in societies dominated by Hinduism or Buddhism is of the devil to accept the reality of energy centers called chakras or meridians as part of the body's design. It is even more difficult for a physician who has completed his or her training to accept the value of nutritional supplements, bioenergetic supports, spinal manipulation, or other "non-conventional" measures to support the body's healing mechanisms. To appreciate the difficulty of keeping an open mind, one must recognize that there are four levels of knowledge one must pass through in mastering any subject.

The Four Levels of Knowledge

The first level of knowledge is that of *unconscious incompetence*. Simply stated, this is the stage at which individuals "don't know that they don't know." A child who has learned to talk may mistakenly believe that he or she can speak to anyone in the world. The child has not yet learned that people speak many different languages. He or she doesn't know what he or she doesn't know.

When a child learns that there are other languages, he or she enters the second phase of learning, the level of *conscious incompetence*. The child now "knows that he or she doesn't know." A child is not particularly threatened by discovering that there is something new to be learned in the area of language. It is simply a matter of recognizing that foreign languages exist. This fact does not threaten the child's self-image or world view. It is simply a new piece of information.

Most Christians are at the first level of knowledge when it comes to understanding the body's design. They accept that the body is comprised of flesh and bone and that it contains various organs. They accept that the body is biochemical and are often anxious to have blood tests performed. They even accept that electrical activity causes the heart to beat and the brain to function, but they have never considered the possibility that disruptions in energy flow or glitches in the body's central computer could be the underlying cause of sickness and aging.

Most physicians are at the first level of knowledge in the fields of nutrition and energetic medicine. They don't know what they don't know. Unlike the case of the child learning that there are other languages in the world, however, the average physician finds it very hard to accept the fact that there are ways of restoring health that he or she has not mastered.

Imagine that you have just invested a total of eleven to fifteen years in preparation for your chosen career. You have completed four years of college, four years of medical school, and three to seven years of post-doctoral residency training to become the best physician you can possibly be. You are taking fifty or more hours of continuing medical education each year to improve your competence. How would you respond if a patient asked you about the benefits of something that had never been mentioned in all your years of training? How would you feel if someone came into your office and said, "Doctor, you need to learn more about nutritional supplementation"? Although the person would mean well, it could be perceived as a threat to your self-image and professional integrity.

The ability of the average physician to accept that there are significant gaps in his or her knowledge and understanding of disease management is further complicated by the demands upon his or her time. Reaching the level of conscious incompetence demands that I either live with the knowledge that I am incompetent or that I take the necessary steps to achieve competence. Imagine that you are a physician spending sixty or more hours per week in the practice of medicine. How would you feel if you suddenly realized that you needed to find time to re-educate yourself? Wouldn't it be easier to reason that you have already learned everything that is known to be of benefit in the prevention and treatment of disease?

Due to the tremendous investment they have made in their medical education and the often overwhelming demands on their time, most physicians will be unable to rise above the level of unconscious incompetence when it comes to healing methods outside of those found in mainstream medical journals and conferences. Ignorance is bliss; knowing that you don't know is torment. Better

4

to take the position that alternative treatment approaches are unresearched, unlikely to be of any benefit, potentially dangerous, and may interfere with standard treatments, than to accept personal incompetence in important aspects of health care and disease management.

When an individual makes a commitment to move forward, the level of *conscious competence* is achieved. This is the level at which people "know, but have to consciously think about what they know." The child who has taken up the challenge of learning a second language will at this stage be able to speak and understand the language, but only by internally translating the words to and from his or her first language. Efforts to speak and understand may be slow and clumsy.

When it comes to disease management, a physician who has moved into the stage of conscious competence will find the flow of the day slowed by the frequent necessity of referring back to reference materials. He or she may become frustrated and abandon the attempt to achieve mastery of the information.

The final level of knowledge is that of *unconscious competence*. At this level an individual "knows what he or she knows." The knowledge flows smoothly, without effort. The child who has reached this level of mastery in a second language can read, listen or speak in that language without needing to internally translate the words. They flow naturally, without effort.

When a physician reaches the level of unconscious competence in modalities that support the body's ability to heal, they will be routinely integrated into any treatment plan. Due to their effectiveness and lack of adverse effects, those modalities will generally become the basis for treatment of any condition. More toxic and aggressive approaches will be reserved for advanced conditions in need of them.

I encourage you to honestly appraise your own level of knowledge in various areas. I believe that it is far better for each of us to admit that we are consciously incompetent in an area than to deny or ridicule its importance. I readily admit that I don't possess the knowledge necessary to make repairs on my car. As a wellness physician I do not possess the ability to perform major surgery. I know almost nothing about drilling for oil and I know that I am not competent to trade commodities.

I believe that it is unrealistic to expect most physicians to become experts in supportive measures. It is not unrealistic to expect those who express a belief in a Creator to be open to learning the true complexity of the human body and be willing to support the healing mechanisms it contains before turning to measures that deny and attack that design under the guise of treatment.

As your knowledge of the design of the human body expands, seek out professionals who are consciously competent to work with the body's design when dealing with health challenges. Avoid physicians or other providers who are unconsciously incompetent. A great deal is known about the design of the human body and the mechanisms that lead to disease and accelerated aging. If a physician says, "We don't know anything about that; it may be dangerous so I don't want you to do it," he or she is demonstrating unconscious incompetence. Seek out a physician who is willing to say, "I don't know much about that, but I'm willing to accept what you know or allow you to consult with someone who does know more about it."

Chapter 2
Crisis Management – Why I Do What I Do

Delight yourself also in the LORD, And He shall give you the desires of your heart.
Commit your way to the LORD, Trust also in Him, And He shall bring it to pass.
–Psalm 37:4-5

On March 1, 1999, I walked away from a successful medical practice that I had worked to establish over the course of twenty years. The decision to do so was the result of three crises that profoundly affected my life. They were a personal health crisis, a personal spiritual crisis, and a crisis in American medicine.

A Personal Health Crisis

In my early forties I found myself in a discomforting position. Throughout my medical career I had often stated, only partly in jest, that mothers and doctors were not allowed to get sick. It is an unwritten law of nature, I would state assuredly. Gradually, however, despite my best efforts to live in denial, my body was forcing me to admit that I was the exception that proved the rule. I was sick!

The thought that I was not the invincible specimen I had always prided myself in being was difficult to accept, but the facts were undeniable. Colds, which had always been rare, were becoming commonplace. Now if my throat became scratchy or sore, I could expect it to progress to bronchitis or pneumonia.

I was tired. My sleep pattern was characterized by waking up as many as six times a night. My wife, Rosalie, complained that I was running in my sleep and kicking her out of the bed. I struggled to wake up each morning and felt as though my head was full of cobwebs. I would plod through the day and plop into an easy chair at night, where I would sit until I raised the energy to climb the stairs and go to bed.

My hands and fingers hurt. I could hold a pen only by keeping my fingers and thumb perfectly straight. I began to wonder if I could continue to see patients, since that entailed writing instructions and prescriptions.

My future appeared dim. My father had died suddenly of a heart attack at age fifty-four. He had been a nonsmoker and physically active. Other male relatives had not fared much better. My cholesterol ratios made it clear that I was doomed to follow the family tradition of dying in the fifth or sixth decade of life. My life expectancy appeared to be down to single digits.

I learned that I did not respond well to the medical treatments I had been taught to administer. I tried numerous medications that were recommended to improve sleep, but they only left me groggier the next day. I took anti-inflammatories for my joint pain, but my stomach became irritated and the joint problem worsened. I tried all the standard cholesterol-lowering medications, but I found that the ones that were the best at improving my numbers caused unbearable muscle pain.

Self-preservation is a powerful motivator. I began to look for answers beyond the established boundaries of my profession. I read what Linus Pauling had written about vitamin C; I read what others were saying about vitamin A, about vitamin E, and about selenium.

I did more than read, however. I began taking vitamin supplements for the first time in my life. I didn't expect anything striking to happen; I was only hoping to stop the hardening of my arteries and avoid having a heart attack at a young age. To my amazement, my joint pain gradually disappeared. This did not occur quickly; the process took place over a period of approximately six months. I now know that this was due to the correction of trace mineral deficiencies in my body by the vitamin/mineral supplement I was taking.

My attitude improved. Only later did I learn of the relationship between B vitamins and a positive mental outlook. I continued to read. I continued to research, expanding my studies to include articles being published in other countries.

I learned that there is more to healthy eating than avoiding fat and adding fiber. I found that supplements beyond basic antioxidants play a role in many aspects of health. One of these, an OPC (oligoproanthocyanidin), finally took away the cobwebs in my head and made it possible for me to sleep restfully and awake alert and refreshed.

Having regained my own health, I could not withhold the information from others. I began to offer those seeking my help nutritional options. Most preferred to stick with symptomatic treatment of their conditions with prescription drugs "because my insurance will pay for it." Some, however, preferred to avoid the drugs and their potential adverse effects and toxicities. As these people began to respond to nutritional supports as I had, I knew that it was time to change my approach to sickness and disease.

A Personal Spiritual Crisis

I was raised in the Christian faith and made a personal commitment to serve Jesus Christ at age nineteen. I felt called to become a physician. I pursued my pre-medical studies at Augsburg College in Minneapolis, Minnesota and was accepted for admission into the University of Minnesota College of Medicine. I graduated in 1972 and subsequently completed a Family Medicine residency at the University of Oklahoma. I entered practice in 1975, providing medical care "from womb to tomb," meaning that I delivered babies, set broken bones, assisted in surgery, treated chronic diseases such as arthritis and diabetes, counseled people with emotional challenges, provided comfort to the dying, and grieved with the survivors.

I attended church regularly and maintained an active prayer life. I recognized that my faith provided a foundation for the ethics upon which I based my practice decisions, but I saw no direct connection between what I believed to be true from a Biblical perspective and how I approached health challenges.

That changed abruptly in 1984 when I met Dr. Carl Baugh, an avid adherent to the Genesis account of creation. As I was confronted with what I believed about the origin of life on earth, I was forced to re-examine my faith and practice.

I had always believed that "in the beginning God created the heavens and the earth," but my education had led me to discount the implications of that statement. College professors and pastors alike had explained that it was enough to believe that God created matter and set the evolutionary process in motion. I had never considered the concept of intelligent design and the implications it held in my approach to maintaining health and addressing disease. Now that I had been forced to face the issue head on, I was facing a crisis of faith.

If I believed that God carefully designed the human body to function in specific ways, I would be forced to admit that what I had been taught in medical school and what I was being taught in my continuing medical education was rooted in error. I would need to face the fact that all of my years of training, all of the hours spent reading peer-reviewed medical journals, and all of the time and money spent to keep current with new drugs and procedures had not prepared me to address the needs of the human body in its battle against disease and aging. I would also run the risk of losing the respect of my peers and the prestige of being a successful medical doctor in my community.

On the other hand, if I wished to maintain my belief that I was a well-trained and competent physician, I would need to reject the idea that a loving Creator had designed the body in a fearful and wonderful way. The decision was too difficult to make at the outset; I placed it on the back burner and managed to successfully avoid making it for several years. Each time the question was raised, however, my inner turmoil intensified.

I could not deny that the complexity of the human entity defies any possibility of having evolved by trial and error, by mere chance. How, for example, did a mother whose immune system is programmed to attack any foreign tissue evolve the ability to carry a baby to term without destroying it? How did that baby evolve the ability to instantly convert its circulatory system from one designed to take oxygen-enriched blood from the placenta to one capable of capturing oxygen from the air sacs of the lungs? How could a single protein molecule have evolved spontaneously, let alone a strand of DNA or a cell capable of reproducing itself?

Finally I was forced to make a choice between my faith and my way of practicing medicine. I chose my faith in a God who designed man in His image over my medical training. As difficult as it would be, I would need to re-educate myself in how to support rather than attack the body in the battle against disease.

Crisis in Medicine

I entered medicine because of a desire to help people who were hurting. I wanted to be able to bind their wounds, treat their illnesses, and be in a position to provide comfort when they faced personal challenges. For a decade, I was privileged to do what I had been called to do.

In the mid 1980s momentous changes in how American medicine was practiced began to take place. The impetus for those changes had been created by the Social Security Act of 1965, which created two governmental programs, Medicare and Medicaid. There were many changes, but they can be summed up in a single word—control.

I entered medicine at a time when doctors were called "physicians" rather than "providers." It was a time when the doctor-patient relationship was considered sacred—as inviolate as the confessional booth. Decisions about care were made within the confines of that relationship. I was able to vary my charges based upon a patient's inability to pay. I could extend professional courtesy to other physicians and members of the clergy.

As time passed, Medicare and Medicaid issued progressively more restrictive and intrusive rules regarding level of payment for services rendered, what diagnostic or therapeutic services were "medically necessary," and what sort of documentation was required to justify payment. Other third parties felt empowered to follow the example being set by government. Health Maintenance Organizations (HMOs) and Preferred Provider Organizations (PPOs) appeared on the scene, each with their own set of rules and restrictions.

The result of the rising control being exercised by third parties resulted in impersonalization. Soon I was no longer considered a caring physician, but a "health care provider" complete with my personal identification number. No longer could I match the personalities of my patients with those of consulting physicians. Instead I was forced to send them to a name on a list of "approved providers," often having no idea of the competency or bedside manner of that individual.

I had always maintained good medical records, but the rise of the third parties turned the emphasis from face-to-face time with the patient to extra time spent documenting each detail of the visit, not to facilitate good medical care, but to satisfy the ever-increasing requirements of those reviewing my charts for evidence to support what I had charged for the visit. The sanctity of the doctor-patient relationship became subjugated to the desire of the third parties to review the charts of their insured. As an "old school" physician, I found it disturbing to watch individuals I did not know indiscriminately thumbing through my patient charts. I had no way of knowing whether they were restricting their review to facts pertinent to billed charges to insured individuals whom they did not know, or whether they were reading sensitive and previously confidential information about a neighbor that they might divulge upon leaving.

I raised the issue to a conservative member of congress during a question and answer session. His response was unexpected, but educational. "The person paying the bill has a right to know everything." I was subsequently informed by the representative of a hospital-based HMO, "We now control 230,000 lives in the Oklahoma City area." He did not say we now *insure* 230,000 lives, but rather we *control* 230,000 lives.

With face-to-face time with my patients limited to that required to listen to their current symptoms and write prescriptions for drugs to relieve them, with diagnostic and therapeutic decisions being dictated by insurance clerks, and with third parties competing for control of people's lives, medical practice was no longer what I had envisioned. The crisis in medicine also dictated that I move on.

Chapter 3

Effective Health Care Reform

Yes, if you cry out for discernment, And lift up your voice for understanding, If you seek her as silver, And search for her as for hidden treasures; Then you will understand the fear of the LORD, And find the knowledge of God. For the LORD gives wisdom; From His mouth come knowledge and understanding . . .
— Proverbs 2:3-6

In 1999, I entered into my personal version of health care reform. It was far different than the congressional health care reform that was a major focus of the first two years of Barack Obama's presidency. The impact that the Affordable Health Care Act of 2010 will have on our society remains to be seen, but one thing is certain. If you wish to optimize your health and maximize the quality and quantity of your life, you must accept personal responsibility for restoring and maintaining your health. To understand why you and you alone hold the keys to true health care reform, you must know what the term "health care" really means.

Understanding the United States' Health Care System

I would like to begin by asking you to imagine that you are traveling in a scenic area. As you reach the crest of a hill, you see before you a tragic situation. People have been inner tubing, canoeing, and rafting down a gently flowing stream, unaware that around a bend in the river, a tributary changes the stream into a raging, churning torrent filled with eddies, undercurrents, and rocks, culminating in a roaring waterfall.

This is a disaster area! People all around are drowning. Some are being battered against the rocks and others are plunging to their death as they pass over the edge of the falls. Attempts, often desperate ones, are being made to rescue them, but as you watch the scene you realize to your horror that this situation has been going on for a long time. Fully organized rescue squads are on the scene. A labyrinth of ropes, buoys and other devices to aid in the rescue effort has been established. In some ways this complicates the problems and pushes people closer to the edge of the falls. As you drive into town, you find that the rescue effort is one of the town's main industries. Rescue schools are in full operation and store after store is selling rescue equipment. The newspapers, radio stations, and television stations have reporters on permanent assignment covering the heroic rescues.

Assessing the situation, you think to yourself, "This is insane . . . Someone has to go upstream and tell people not to put in." But when you arrive upstream you find another town that has entire industries devoted to recreational use of the river. Stores there are selling tubes, rafts and canoes; promotional efforts encouraging people to enter the water are all around. Billboards display the joy of the float trip; radio spots and television ads have catchy jingles urging people to get on their way. It's a real carnival atmosphere!

You begin to tell people about the dangers involved in floating the river, but most of them jump in anyway, and when you suggest that they should at least wear a life vest, many laugh and quote local experts who have assured them that it isn't necessary and would be a waste of money.

If what I have just described sounds like a nightmare, it is. But in reality, it is an allegory of what is called the United States Health Care System. The system isn't designed to keep people well; it is designed to rescue them when they get into trouble. This country does have one of the best disease care systems in the world, but far too many people are finding themselves in the midst of a medical crisis. At times, although well intentioned, the rescue system actually has unwanted side effects that make people get worse or even die.

Additionally, we don't have an active disease prevention system in this country; we have a disease promotion system. Just like the town that was tied to the industries sending people into the river, our economy is heavily dependent upon industries that send people down the road to illness. Some of them, I think, are obvious, such as the tobacco and the liquor industries, but some are not so obvious. Major food suppliers, nonalcoholic beverage industries, and manufacturers of toxic personal care items and cleaning supplies do the same. All are selling people down the river. Consider the top ten grossing items in United States grocery stores. The grocery store is where you go to get nutritious things, right? Number 1 on the list is Marlboro cigarettes; number 2 is Coca Cola Classic; number 3 is Pepsi Cola; number 4 is Kraft processed cheese; number 5 is Diet Coke; number 6 is Campbell's soup; number 7 is Budweiser beer; number 8 is Tide detergent; number 9 is Folger's coffee; and number 10 is Winston cigarettes.

What "Preventive Medicine" Really Means

We really don't have true preventive medicine in this country. Most of what passes for prevention is really early detection. A mammogram can't prevent breast cancer, it can only help find cancers in earlier stages of development, and a PSA test can't prevent prostate cancer, it can only suggest that a tumor is present. Wouldn't you rather decrease your chances of developing a disease than simply hope to catch it in an earlier stage?

What is called preventive medicine is really simply trying to prevent a more serious disease from developing. Treating high blood pressure with medications may help prevent strokes, but why aren't we trying to prevent the high blood pressure in the first place? Lowering cholesterol levels with drugs may decrease the risk of a heart attack, but wouldn't it make more sense to prevent the changes in blood vessels and LDL cholesterol that actually cause the problem?

The Danger of Treating Symptoms

Because the United States Health Care System does not place a high value on time spent listening to people and thoroughly evaluating their issues, most general physicians and many sub-specialists are forced to schedule patient visits at ten to fifteen minute intervals. Of that, actual face-to-face time is often limited to three or four minutes. This is sufficient only to listen to the primary symptoms that are present and write a prescription for a medication that will relieve those symptoms.

Treating symptoms is an extremely dangerous approach to health challenges. Symptoms are the body's warning signals, comparable to the warning lights on a car's dashboard. Suppose you are driving down the highway when you glance down and notice a red light on the dashboard that says "oil." At that point you have several options. You may try to ignore the light and keep driving. Unfortunately, the light keeps attracting your attention so you pull over. The average person would call for assistance, but you are more creative. You find a pair of pliers in the trunk, raise the hood, identify the wire leading to the annoying light, and clip it. You restart the vehicle, look down, breathe a sigh of relief that the irritating light is no longer shining, and drive on.

At this point you are probably saying, "That's crazy! I would never do *that*. My engine could burn up before I reached my destination." You are absolutely correct in your thinking, but millions of people take drugs to block symptoms every day. Headache, heartburn, cough, and tiredness are examples of body warning lights. Pain relievers, acid-blockers, cough suppressants, and power drinks are means of clipping the wires. The symptoms will disappear for a time, but, just as in the case of a vehicle with a clipped oil light, a major breakdown is likely to occur somewhere down the road.

A Different Approach to Health Challenges

I spent thirty years of my life working in the disease care system. I've seen incredible technical advances over that period of time. I've witnessed the advent of CAT scanners, MRIs, organ transplants, laser surgery, angioplasties, and artificial joint replacements—just to name a few. Over the years, however, I've become convinced that the answer to the health challenges faced by the vast majority of people is not high tech—it is low tech. It is simply providing the body with the basic support it needs to function properly while decreasing exposure to substances or energies that attack or break down the body's defenses.

My personal health challenges drove me to look for answers beyond those recommended in standard medical textbooks and mainstream medical journals. As my personal health improved, I felt compelled to share what I had learned with those seeking my assistance in dealing with their health challenges.

I whispered a prayer: "God, if you will teach me how to help people truly get well rather than just treat symptoms, I will look at anything and everything, no matter how strange it sounds to my medically trained ears. If, after careful study, I am confident that it cannot cause any harm and I can, to my personal satisfaction, understand the mechanism by which it produces results, I will offer it to those seeking my help."

For nearly two decades I have been asking the question, "What else is out there that I don't know about?" For nearly two decades I have been finding answers. It has been, and continues to be, a grand and glorious adventure. I invite you to join me in that adventure by not only reading about the answers I have found, but taking steps to implement them in your own life. I invite you to engage in true health care reform.

Chapter 4

A Philosophy of Wellness

Beloved, I pray that you may prosper in all things and be in health,
just as your soul prospers.
— 3 John 1:2

As a physician, I had been educated to think in terms of sickness. When someone became ill they would come to me for treatment. I was not taught how to improve a person's level of wellness, only how to deal with their sickness. I had not been taught how to keep people out of the river. As I embarked on my new career as a "wellness physician," it was essential that I understand the meaning of true wellness.

The Health Continuum

Wellness is the opposite of sickness. If sickness is defined as a disordered, weakened, or unsound condition, wellness can be defined as an ordered, strengthened, and sound condition. Sickness and wellness are polar opposites, and there is a vast distance between manifest sickness and optimum wellness. They are at opposite ends of the spectrum of health, as illustrated in figure 1.

Figure 1	The Health Continuum
Sickness _____ Wellness	

Being well is quite different from not being sick. As I was explaining this concept to a group of individuals a man made this comment: "You're absolutely right! I had my heart attack at 8:02 on a Thursday morning. I didn't realize it at the time, but I wasn't perfectly well at 8:01."

The gentlemen *felt* well at 8:01. He *thought* he was well at 8:01. In actuality, he was very sick—the time bomb that was ticking in his diseased coronary arteries was seconds away from exploding.

The condition of one's health is never stagnant. At any point in time an individual is either moving to the left or the right on the health continuum line. He or she is either losing ground in the battle against disease or advancing toward optimum wellness, which I define as the state at which body, soul, and spirit are in harmony and the body's healing mechanisms are operating at peak efficiency.

Defining Sickness and Wellness

It is important to understand that sickness and wellness cannot be determined accurately by observing a person's physical condition. A person who appears to be in robust health may actually be very, very sick. The man who related the story about his heart attack is an example.

A few years ago, Rosalie and I met a friend for lunch. He looked great and he told us that he was feeling the best he had ever felt in his life. He did not know and we did not suspect that a deadly cancer was silently advancing within his body. It was discovered shortly after our visit. He died less than three months later. Although he was extremely sick, he believed himself to be in the best condition possible.

On the other hand, an individual may have a debilitating condition but be functioning in the range of optimum wellness. Someone who is known to have cancer, but who has instituted the changes necessary to engage his or her body's innate healing ability would be in this category. The same would be true of a paraplegic who is at peace with his or her condition and who is following basic wellness principles.

It is important to consider ways of moving toward wellness on a day to day basis. Perhaps that will mean changing an eating habit. It may mean altering activity level. It could involve adding a nutritional support, switching to a non-toxic cleaning product in the kitchen, or decreasing the amount of time spent listening to the news. Optimum wellness is not a destination; it is a quest. Daily choices determine how successful the search will be.

The Lethargy/Vitality Scale

A second indicator of health status is the lethargy/vitality scale. This is different from the sickness/wellness scale. While the sickness/wellness continuum is largely physical in nature, the lethargy/vitality continuum describes an individual's emotional or spiritual state.

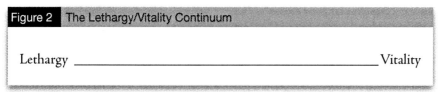

Figure 2   The Lethargy/Vitality Continuum

Lethargy _____ Vitality

People who rank high on the vitality scale are enthusiastic about life. They are excited about what each day has to offer. Their energy level is high and they are optimistic. A normal child is a great example of someone operating high on the vitality scale.

In contrast, people at the other extreme are lethargic. Nothing excites them. Those who are the most lethargic have decided that things are never going to get better, so they are simply going through the motions of living.

Wellness Quadrants

Used together, the sickness/wellness and lethargy/vitality scales can provide tremendous insight into an individual's state of health. This is shown in figure 3.

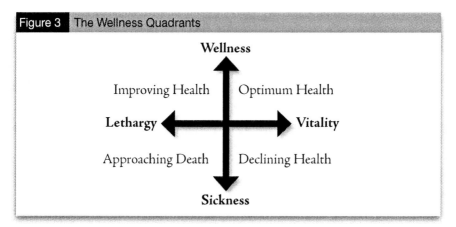

Figure 3   The Wellness Quadrants

An individual who is functioning at a high level of wellness and vitality is achieving optimum health. The goal of each of us should be to operate within the right upper quadrant of the diagram.

The man who related his experience prior to a heart attack and our friend who appeared so healthy just before he learned that he had an advanced cancer are examples of people who are functioning in the right lower quadrant. Their health is declining. They are sick, even though they feel well and appear to be in good health.

A person who has recognized that a challenge exists because of loss of vitality, but who has implemented changes that will result in moving toward wellness, is in the left upper quadrant. Over time he or she should regain vitality and move to the right upper quadrant.

Individuals who are in the process of dying are those in the left lower quadrant. They are sick and know that this is the case. Rather than engaging in behaviors that have the potential of moving forward, they continue to eat what they have always eaten. They continue to pursue the same daily activities they have always pursued. As their disease advances and their vitality wanes, they lose hope and simply go through the motions of living.

Unfortunately, the end does not always come quickly. The world is full of people who died in their thirties and weren't buried until their seventies or eighties.

The goal of this book is to give you the knowledge required to move to the outermost point of the right upper quadrant in the health diagram. It is to empower you to live life to the fullest and to keep your intrinsic God-given healing mechanisms working at peak efficiency.

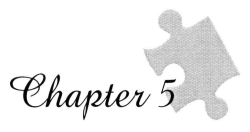

Chapter 5

Treat Your Body like a Palace, Not a Garbage Dump

For no one ever hated his own flesh, but nourishes and cherishes it,
just as the Lord does the church.
– Ephesians 5:29

Pursuing Wellness

Health is not a static condition. Each minute of every day we are either moving toward wellness or we are heading for sickness. The decisions we make day-by-day, week-by-week, and year-by-year have consequences. Some are immediately apparent, but most appear many years later.

We live in a society in which people desire immediate gratification. Because symptoms demand attention, many find it appealing and gratifying to treat them when they appear. Few find it satisfying to pursue wellness, because progress is often apparent only after months or years rather than in minutes or days.

Even as a wellness physician most of my time is spent addressing the signs and symptoms of disease, for it is only when illness presents that the average individual begins to seek the health that has been lost. Over the years I have observed that how a person treats his or her body often determines whether or not a disease will appear and how effectively the body will rise to the challenge if a disease appears. The unfortunate truth is that most people give more thought to what they choose to throw into the trash can than what is allowed to enter or come in contact with their bodies.

The principles involved in treating the body well are simple ones. Perhaps this is one of the reasons so many physicians choose to pursue diagnoses and treat symptoms rather than promote wellness. Learning the intricacies of hundreds of diseases and thousands of symptoms, each with a specific treatment, is intellectually challenging. On the surface, teaching people to respect their bodies seems quite elementary, and unworthy of someone with eleven to fifteen years of formal training.

This is a false perception. Understanding the subtleties of basic principles and the intricate way in which those variables affect the body's ability to maintain and restore health is a never-ending quest. The pursuit of wellness is the pursuit of a lifetime.

Breathe Clean Air

Most people give almost no thought to air quality. Nothing seems to be more taken for granted than breathing when the respiratory system is working well. Poor air quality can damage the lungs and bronchial tubes, making it difficult or impossible to take a satisfying breath. When that occurs it is no longer possible to take breathing for granted, for nothing is more desperately sought than a good breath when the body is short of oxygen. Unfortunately, by the time someone becomes notably short of breath it is often too late; irreversible damage has already been done.

What consideration is given to air quality usually relates to the outdoor air quality as defined by the Environmental Protection Agency. A high pollen count or an ozone alert is a cause for concern, but the air quality within our control affects us to a much greater extent than the air that is outside of our personal control.

Having never smoked, I have great difficulty empathizing with those who choose to do so. It is difficult for me to imagine voluntarily breathing hot noxious gases on a regular basis. Nothing influences personal air quality to a greater extent than the decision to smoke cigarettes, cigars, or pipes.

Neither do I feel any sympathy for those who argue that governmental restrictions on smoking in public areas are an invasion of privacy. Even if one assumes that each person has a fundamental right to destroy his or her health, it cannot be asserted that they have the right to adversely affect the health of others.

Personal air quality is adversely affected in other ways. The introduction of toxic fumes into the home is quite commonplace. People routinely purchase and use household cleaners that emit harmful gases. Room deodorizers are commonly used even though most simply "cover" odors by overwhelming the body's sense of smell.

I have needed to hospitalize individuals who have been overcome by fumes while cleaning a confined space such as a shower or bathroom, but the body can be damaged when using such products in open areas as well. A man once consulted me regarding a cough that had been present for two weeks. We determined that the cough had been triggered by inhaling naphthalene in his home after his wife had scattered mothballs around the outside walls of the house to repel pests.

Personal air quality can be adversely affected, but it can also be improved by taking the proper steps. A mask or approved respirator should be used when performing tasks that generate airborne dust or fumes. Farmers, miners, and welders, for example, can decrease their occupational risk of lung disease by wearing approved devices when air quality is poor. Hobbyists as well as professionals should wear masks when sanding or spray-painting articles.

Indoor air quality is often far worse than that outside homes and offices. The EPA estimates that the air inside homes and offices contains chemicals at levels up to seventy times that of outdoor air, and that overall indoor air pollution is five to ten times worse than that of outdoor air.[1] Dust mites, animal dander, molds, and other particulates are typically present. Levels of carbon monoxide, carbon dioxide, sulfur dioxide, and nitrogen oxides from cooking and heating fuels can reach dangerously high levels. Carpets, paneling, and insulation can infuse formaldehyde and other chemicals into the home environment for years after installation.

Unlike the outside air, which is periodically cleansed by falling rain, the air inside most buildings is not freshened automatically. It is necessary to take specific steps to improve and maintain indoor air quality.

It is important to service or replace filters in the home's ventilation system regularly. Electrostatic air filters should be considered, as they are able to remove more than 90 percent of the fungi, mold, lint, animal hair and dander, pollen, dust, smoke, and other particles from the circulating air, a much higher percentage than is removed by disposable fiber filters.

Air purification units are also available. Many options exist, but there is one constant: no air purifier will work well through walls. Air purification will be far better if smaller units are used in multiple locations than when one large unit is purchased based on the square footage of the entire house.

Controlling the humidity of the air is important, particularly in the winter when the indoor air is being heated. Indoor air in heated homes is often drier than the air in Death Valley. This is very irritating to the membranes lining the respiratory tract. Dry air can cause nosebleeds, cracked lips, and predispose people to colds and other infections.

Simply placing a teapot or pan of water on the stove is woefully inadequate to humidify winter air. A humidifier of proper capacity should be used. It is important that it be cleaned regularly to prevent the growth of mold, which, if present, will be blown into the air and become a health risk.

Avoid Carbonated Beverages

Water is one of the body's greatest needs. I sometimes refer to pure water as *the* essential nutrient. Unfortunately, water is not the beverage of choice for many people. Carbonated beverages are the most commonly consumed beverages in the United States today. Children are introduced to them at an early age. I have seen infants and toddlers sucking on baby bottles that contain not milk or water but soda.

I remember my first soft drink. It was a most unpleasant experience. The fizz bubbled into my nose and the fluid burned as it passed through my esophagus. My instinct was to never drink something like that again, but the peer pressure of my cousins and the steady exposure to Coca-Cola ads caused me to persevere until I could not only tolerate sodas, but came to crave them as the only acceptable fluid to drink.

I was fortunately able to kick the habit about twenty years ago. Several years after doing so, I couldn't resist touring *The World of Coke* during a trip to Atlanta. Coca-Cola is arguably the world's most recognizable trademark. It's not surprising that Coca-Cola is a $100 billion corporation.

The tour ended in two tasting rooms. One was lined with spouts that spewed domestic recipes like Coca-Cola Classic, Tab, Mountain Dew, and Fresca, while the other offered international blends.

One sip of the real thing was enough to remind me why I had come to prefer pure water. The thick syrupy texture was nauseating, and the carbonation burned as it passed down my throat.

Beverages, like foods, are an acquired taste. If any proof of this was needed, watching the faces of visitors as they sampled one of the international brews was ample evidence. The concoction, a big seller in its country of origin—I won't say which one so as not to rob you of the opportunity of discovering it for yourself should you ever visit *The World of Coke*—had a very distinctive flavor that can best be described as eau d' dead skunk.

The difference in people's taste for beverages would be a mere curiosity, were it not for the tragic consequences that result from imbibing the sugary, fizzy drinks. Sodas may one day be recognized as rivaling tobacco products in their adverse effects on health. The phosphoric and carbonic acids that produce the "fizz" have an extremely negative impact on health and wellness.

The most well-documented hazard of drinking soft drinks is the damage done to tooth enamel. Cola-type beverages cause erosions on tooth surfaces, which predispose teeth to decay.[2] The effect is less pronounced if the beverage is consumed quickly, and more damaging if it is sipped slowly allowing the liquid to remain in contact with the teeth for a longer period of time. Unfortunately, sodas are sipped in the majority of instances.

Sugar-containing soft drinks are playing a role in the increasing incidence of obesity in our society. Each 12-ounce serving contains 140 calories and 39 grams of sugar. A Harvard study of the eating, drinking, and exercise habits of children revealed that for every soft drink consumed per day, the risk of obesity increased by 50 percent.[3] This is highly significant, given that one out of every three children in the United States is now considered obese.

The highly acidic drinks have also been shown to weaken bones and increase the risk of developing osteoporosis.[4,5] This is because the pH (acidity) of phosphoric acid is 2.8, but that of the blood is 7.4. A drop in blood pH to 7.2 is life threatening. The significance of this quickly becomes apparent when one considers that each 1-point drop in pH represents a tenfold increase in acidity. That means that a substance with a pH of 2.8 is nearly 100,000 times more acidic than human blood!

When a soft drink is consumed, the body must neutralize the acid it contains or death will ensue. Acid neutralization is accomplished by pulling minerals from soft tissues and ultimately from the storehouse, which is bone. In past decades, osteoporotic fractures occurred primarily in elderly women who had lost bone after going through menopause. In 2000, however, a study of teenaged girl athletes found that cola drinkers were nearly five times more likely to sustain a fracture than girls who did not drink carbonated beverages.[6]

The acids also break down beneficial nutrients before they can be absorbed and utilized in the body. This is why club soda works so well to remove fruit juice stains from carpets. In addition, the high sugar content of regular soft drinks destroys the effectiveness of the immune system, and the effect of long-term consumption of aspartame, saccharin, or sucralose in "diet" drinks has never been fully evaluated. Several studies have demonstrated that soft drinks in general and colas in particular cause changes that promote the development of kidney stones.[7] People with a history of kidney stones should be advised to avoid carbonated beverages.

Soft drinks are commonly sold in aluminum cans. Aluminum, a toxic metal, leaches out of the container and into the beverage. This point was driven home to me one day when I was given an aluminum can containing water during an airline flight. The strong metallic taste of the water made it undrinkable, but the strong flavor of carbonated beverages masks any metal they may contain. Aluminum is one of the metals, along with lead, mercury and iron, suspected of participating in the steps leading to Alzheimer's disease. Deposition of aluminum in muscles may be one of the factors that influence the course of fibromyalgia.

To be fair, a number of studies, supported in many cases by grants from the soft drink industry, conclude that neither regular nor diet sodas have any effect upon health and can and should be included in the daily diet. Having lived through the era of tobacco institute studies that failed to demonstrate any adverse effect from smoking, I'm unimpressed. I'll stick with logic.

Drink Pure Water

With the exception of oxygen, water is the most critical and essential nutrient in the human body. Deprived of oxygen, we will die within a matter of minutes. Deprived of water, we will die in a matter of days.

Water makes up 70 percent of our body weight. Without the presence of water, our cells and tissues would collapse. Without water, nutrients could not be absorbed and transported to our individual cells. Without water, toxic wastes could not be transported from our cells to the pores of our skin or to our kidneys, nor could they be excreted by these organs. Without water, life would be impossible.

Lack of adequate water intake creates a wide variety of symptoms. An individual may feel dizzy and lightheaded, especially when changing positions. Muscle aching is common. Often, as dehydration progresses, nausea develops, which worsens the situation by discouraging necessary intake. Lack of adequate water intake predisposes to dry, irritated skin, constipation, headaches, kidney stones, salivary duct stones, urinary tract infections, sinus and bronchial infections, bloating, and fatigue. Inadequate water intake results in a thickening of the blood, which increases the risk of heart attack and stroke. Lack of adequate water intake is one of the leading causes of premature aging.

A common question is, "How much water should I be drinking?" While various rules such as "six to eight glasses a day" are sometimes given, I find these inadequate. The amount of water required while sitting quietly on a cool rainy day is vastly different than that required while working in the yard on a hot summer day. When my daughters and I hiked the Grand Canyon, we were advised, "Any canteen smaller than a gallon is a toy!"

So how much water should you be drinking? I recommend following the advice of the body itself. You should regularly drink enough water to keep your urine pale. An added step is to drink 16 ounces of water over a 15 minute period in the mid-morning and again in the mid-afternoon. This flushes the system with water and aids in detoxifying the system as well as maintaining optimum hydration of the tissues. I often have an individual say, "I can't get my urine pale because I take vitamins that turn my urine yellow." This is not true. If water intake is adequate, the urine will be a very pale yellow rather than a deep, bright yellow, despite the presence of B vitamins in the urine.

What type of water should be drunk? Let me begin by saying that it is unlikely that any source of naturally pure water exists today. All water should be purified before it is allowed to enter the body. I highly recommend that a reverse osmosis water purification system be purchased for the home. When buying bottled water it is important that the label state that the water was purified by distillation or reverse osmosis. The term "natural spring water" is meaningless. Since a portion of my city's water supply comes from an underground aquifer, I could fill gallon jugs from my kitchen tap and legally sell them as "Spring Water."

I am dismayed by the number of people and organizations that are promoting consumption of tap water today. The argument that bottled water is really tap water misses the point. Yes, suppliers of products like Aquafina, Dasani, and others begin with tap water, but the end product is the result of multiple purification procedures. To suggest that purified bottled water is tap water is akin to saying that tap water is sewer water, since tap water begins as sewer water before being treated to remove most disease-causing organisms.

Tap water is not healthy for children and other living things. Municipalities produce "potable" water, which meets certain criteria set by the EPA as safe for consumption. Most potable water is not free of toxic chemicals. Each quarter I receive a water quality report from my city's water department. The report lists dozens of chemicals that are present in the water and proudly proclaims that they have been kept within acceptable limits. This simply means that water containing low levels of toxins is unlikely to cause immediate illness when drunk. Unfortunately, the long-term consequences of drinking water that contains small amounts of those chemicals are unknown. Just because we don't have an outbreak of diarrhea doesn't mean that there isn't a problem.

Because it is necessary to kill disease-causing organisms in the water, chlorine or similar chemicals are usually added. Chlorine is a deadly poison. Chlorine gas was used as a weapon in World War I. As little as 0.085 percent chlorine in the atmosphere causes death in a few minutes. Each bottle of household chlorine bleach states KEEP OUT OF REACH OF CHILDREN and carries the following: "WARNING: Hazardous to humans and domestic animals. Causes substantial but temporary eye injury. Do not get in eyes or on clothing. Harmful if swallowed. May irritate skin. For prolonged use, wear gloves."

Chlorine is added to water supplies to kill living organisms. Your body is a living organism. In addition, your body is designed to rely upon living bacteria in your intestinal tract to aid with food digestion and production of B vitamins. Does chlorine stop killing bacteria when you drink it? No! It continues to kill, eliminating most of the normal flora, the bacteria needed for optimum health, in your intestinal tract.

I believe that people should drink water purified by reverse osmosis filtration or, if that is unavailable, distilled water. Those processes eliminate the toxins and dangerous organisms from the water and produce pure, refreshing water for human consumption. Minerals may be added for taste. It is amazing how many non-water drinkers suddenly become habitual water drinkers when they experience the satisfaction of drinking pure water. If an individual still resists drinking water, it may be sweetened by adding a small amount of fruit juice or consumed as an herbal or green tea.

Beverages such as coffee and black tea have a diuretic effect, which means that they encourage elimination of water from the body. Therefore, they can actually promote mild dehydration. Most soft drinks have the same effect.

Water is best consumed at room temperature. A standard treatment for a bleeding ulcer is to rinse the stomach with ice water. Ice water causes the blood vessels in the stomach to constrict, which is beneficial if one wishes to stop bleeding, but is detrimental if one is hoping to digest food efficiently.

Use a Shower Filter

There is an aspect of water usage that is vitally important but commonly ignored. Read the warning from the container of chlorine bleach once more. It states that chlorine may cause eye injury and irritate the skin. Since this is true, does it make any sense to shower with chlorinated water? Filters for showerheads are available. These remove chlorine and other volatile chemicals. I have seen many skin conditions improve when a shower filter has been put into use. My wife, Rosalie, is an example of this. She suffered from itchy red blotches on her skin from the day she left the farm (where no chemicals had been added to the water) to the day we installed a shower filter.

I have had observant people tell me that they feel tired after taking a shower. There is a logical explanation for this. One evening I was having dinner with a group that included Fred Van Liew, President of Essential Water and Air in Dallas, Texas. One of the people at the table asked Fred why he recommended the use of shower filters. Fred turned to me and asked, "Don't doctors sometimes prescribe medications as patches that are applied to the skin?"

"Yes," I replied.

"How big are those patches?" asked Fred.

"Usually about the size of a quarter," I answered.

"So," Fred continued, "it's possible to give an entire day's drug dosage by applying it to a spot on the skin no larger than a quarter?"

"Yes," I confirmed, "sometimes one patch can supply the dosage needed for an entire week."

Fred then explained to the questioner that the skin is highly absorbent. Not only can drugs be absorbed through the skin, but chemicals in shower water can also be absorbed. He pointed out that it is possible to take in more chlorine and other chemicals during a brief shower than one could possibly ingest by drinking the water throughout the day. It is this load of chemicals that can cause transient tiredness following a shower.

The Value of Water Catalysts

Drinking purified water and showering or bathing in filtered water are fundamental steps in slowing the aging process, but they are only the basic measures that can be taken to improve water quality. It is possible to do much more. To understand how it is possible and why it is important to enhance drinking water, it is necessary to recognize the true nature of water.

Chemistry teaches that the formula for water is H_2O; it is a molecule that consists of one oxygen atom bound to two hydrogen atoms. While this is true, what is rarely said is that water never appears as individual H_2O molecules in the environment. If it did, it would boil at 223.15 Kelvin (minus 58 degrees Fahrenheit) and freeze at 173.15 Kelvin (minus 148 degrees Fahrenheit). This is referred to as a phase anomaly; it is believed to be due to bonds between the hydrogen atoms in water molecules. It is this hydrogen bonding that causes the water to form clusters. The fact that water is made up of clusters rather than individual H_2O molecules explains why it is possible to fill a water glass above the brim without spilling the water. Pouring water slowly into the glass is akin to stacking marbles. The clusters (marbles) can extend above the top of the glass without spilling over.

Clusters give water many of its unique properties, but when the average cluster size is large, the ability of water to pass through cell membranes is compromised. This makes it more difficult to carry nutrients into and remove toxins from the cells of the body.

A number of catalysts capable of breaking water clusters into smaller sizes have been developed. One of the first was created by Dr. John Willard, a professor at the South Dakota School of Mines. Dr. Willard initially developed his water catalyst as a means to improve the extraction of coal and for use as a degreaser. What Dr. Willard had discovered, in actuality, was a simple method for breaking some of the hydrogen bonds in water clusters. By adding an ounce of his catalyst to a gallon of water, it is possible to significantly improve the hydrating capacity of the water and to erase much of its memory. Several variations on Dr. Willard's original recipe have proven to be effective in reducing cluster size.

An additional factor to be considered in producing water that is optimized for drinking is the amount of energy it contains. Molecules are able to capture and store energy as the bonds between the atoms are stretched and relaxed. Since our bodies are made up of atoms and molecules, logic suggests that the energy of the body will be affected by the amount of energy captured and stored in its atoms and molecules.

The most abundant molecule in the body is H_2O. Water molecules make up 70 percent of our body weight. The brain is 75 percent water, blood is almost 95 percent water, and our bones are nearly 25 percent water. This being the case, the amount of energy contained in the water molecules of our bodies will have a major impact on total energy stores.

Water is an amazing substance. Chemically, it is made up of two hydrogen atoms attached to one oxygen atom by means of a "covalent" bond. The hydrogen atoms are separated by 104 degrees. As the temperature of the water rises and falls, this angle is stretched and relaxed, an action that causes the water molecule to capture energy.

In nature, water not only undergoes changes in temperature; it also forms eddies, or vortices, as it flows. This spinning action also adds energy to the water molecules. Exposure to natural or man-made electromagnetic fields will also affect the amount of energy stored in water.

Water is an excellent solvent, capable of holding many other substances in solution. It is also magnetic, having positive and negative poles. Magnetic Resonance Imaging machines (MRIs) are able to provide a detailed picture of the inner anatomy of the body through the use of a powerful magnetic field that aligns the water molecules in the body.

Because of its solvent and magnetic properties, water possesses the ability to remember vibratory frequencies, much in the same manner as voice or musical vibrations can be captured and remembered on magnetic recording tape. This means that even though substances such as chlorine or other dissolved solids have been removed by filtration or distillation, the water still retains a record of them. This vibratory record may be transferred to other systems including living organisms. It has been demonstrated that the temperature at which water is able to release or acquire the greatest amount of information is 37.5 decrees centigrade or 98.6 degrees Fahrenheit, the precise temperature of the human body.[8]

Using devices that are capable of measuring the excitement of electrons or other particles, scientists have been able to measure the inherent energy in substances or systems. Using a scale referred to as the "Biophoton" or "Bovis" scale, the innate energy level can be recorded and compared to that of other systems.

The Bovis scale ranges from zero to infinity. The neutral point for the human body is 6,500. Energy levels above 6,500 are therefore life enhancing or life supporting, while energies below 6,500 are life depleting.

Most water tested today measures between 2,000 and 5,000 Bovis. This means that we face a dilemma. When we drink water, as we must, our body must provide energy to bring that water up to life standards. This places an energy drain on the system. While we are being nourished biochemically, we are being depleted biophysically. Is it any wonder that so many people feel so tired so often?

Modern water catalysts such as *Quanta Water* not only lower cluster size, but enhance the water's energy. Devices such as the *Vitalizer Plus* duplicate the mechanics that renew and energize water in nature. Providing microclustered, harmonically balanced, energized water to the body is one of the main steps that can be taken to restore and maintain health.

Eat a Wellness Diet

To grow and remain healthy, our bodies require nutrients, constituents in food that provide building blocks for maintenance and repair. Three major substances—fat, protein, and carbohydrate—are found in the foods that we eat. They are referred to as "macronutrients." Other important constituents such as vitamins and minerals are called "micronutrients."

Each macronutrient plays important roles in the body. It is important to understand some of these when making dietary choices.

Proteins

Protein is comprised of amino acids. The body needs amino acids to manufacture enzymes, hormones, and, of course, proteins. Proteins are an important component of every cell. Hair and nails are comprised almost exclusively of protein, and protein is an important building block of bone, muscle, cartilage, skin, and even blood. Protein is also needed to repair damaged tissues.

The amount of protein required to perform these functions is grossly overestimated by most individuals. A common myth among bodybuilders says that extra protein is required to build muscle mass, but this is not the case. Active men and teenage boys require more protein than other groups, but all of their needs can be met with only seven ounces of protein daily. Most people, including older children, teenagers, active women, and sedentary men, do well with six ounce of protein daily. Young children, sedentary women, and seniors need only five ounces.

The wide variety of protein sources are also unappreciated by many. "Where do you get your protein?" is almost always the first question asked when someone learns that I rarely eat meat. The answer is that legumes, nuts, and whole grains are rich sources of high-quality protein. Ounce for ounce, legumes and nuts provide as much protein as beef or poultry. Whole grain products, such as whole wheat bread, provide about half the protein per ounce.

Proteins are not created equal, however. When animal protein is digested and metabolized an acidic ash is created, which must be neutralized. The body uses minerals such as calcium to accomplish this. Therefore, diets high in animal protein promote the development of osteoporosis over time as minerals are pulled from the bone to maintain a normal pH in the blood. When plant proteins break down an alkaline (non-acidic) residue is created. Alkaline environments are associated with a lower incidence of cancer, osteoporosis, and degenerative diseases such as arthritis.

Fats

Fats give texture and flavor to food, and they provide a greater feeling of satiety than proteins and carbohydrates. The low-fat diet craze that preceded the low-carb approach resulted in a significant increase in obesity rates. People who restricted their fat intake were found to be eating more calories because they did not experience "fullness" as quickly. Fats are also needed for the absorption of fat-soluble vitamins including A, D, E, and K. The body uses fats to manufacture anti-inflammatory compounds, cell membranes, and brain chemicals. Fats are needed to maintain healthy skin and hair and for a host of other maintenance tasks.

Different fats, like different proteins, behave differently. Most saturated fats, which are solid at room temperature, increase the risk of atherosclerosis and promote inflammation. Exceptions are vegetable fats found in foods such as avocado and coconut, which actually provide health benefits. Certain unsaturated fats, which are liquid at room temperature, lower the risk of atherosclerosis, enable the body to produce anti-inflammatory compounds, and manufacture cell membranes appropriately. The role of specific unsaturated fats will be explained in Chapter Seven.

Carbohydrates

Carbohydrates, although much maligned in recent years, are also essential to good health. Carbohydrates provide energy and increase our ability to perform prolonged activity. They are the primary energy source in the brain and as such enhance mental performance. Carbohydrates are needed to restore energy stores in muscles after activity and they increase the body's ability to build muscle mass. They are essential to maintenance of blood sugar levels and free proteins for use in the areas in which they are needed.

Like proteins and fats, carbohydrates are available in different forms. Simple carbohydrates, sometimes referred to as simple sugars, are generally found in fruits. Complex carbohydrates, which are made up of starches and fibers, are found primarily in vegetables. While some have attempted to define simple carbohydrates as "bad" and complex carbohydrates as "good," both types provide distinct benefits. Far more important than the distinction of simple or complex is the question of the source of the carbohydrate.

Whole foods (fruits, vegetables, and whole grains) typically contain a combination of simple and complex carbohydrates. In many cases, fats and proteins are also present. Refined and processed foods (white rice, white flour, white sugar, candy bars, sodas, etc.) are typically high in simple sugars without the fiber, vitamins, and minerals found in whole foods.

A simple carbohydrate eaten as part of a whole food behaves much differently than when it is consumed alone. The disparity can be seen by comparing the glycemic index of a food with its glycemic load. All carbohydrates affect blood glucose levels. The degree to which a food influences blood sugar is determined by comparing it to the effect of pure glucose. Glucose is given a value of 100 on the glycemic index. While knowing a food's glycemic index is somewhat helpful, recognizing its glycemic load, which is defined as the effect of a typical serving, is much more revealing.

The humble carrot provides an excellent example of the difference between a food's glycemic index and its glycemic load. Carrots were initially reported to have a glycemic index of 92, causing people to believe that eating a carrot affects the blood sugar nearly as greatly as eating pure sugar. It has since been discovered that the glycemic index of carrots is closer to 47.

The glycemic load of eating a serving of raw or cooked carrots is only 3. This is because the starch and fiber within the carrot limit the amount of carrot sugar that can be consumed at one time. In contrast, carrot juice carries a glycemic load of 10 and a carrot muffin a glycemic load of 20!

To put this in perspective, it is currently believed that a total daily glycemic load of 160 or greater is associated with a significantly increased risk of developing diabetes. To remain in good health over one's lifetime, it is advisable to keep the glycemic load of one's daily diet to 100 or less. This means that an individual could safely eat the equivalent of thirty-three servings of raw or cooked carrots each day, but only five carrot muffins over the course of a day. One would not limit one's diet to carrots, of course, but this example points out the dramatic difference in glycemic load between carbohydrates in the form of whole vegetables and foods containing refined carbohydrates. It would be nearly impossible to reach a daily glycemic load of 100 by eating vegetables alone.

Fruits show a similar pattern. Fresh strawberries, for example, carry a glycemic load of 1, while that of strawberry jam is 10. A whole orange has a glycemic load of 3, but orange juice a value of 12. Most fruits produce a glycemic load of 3 to 7. Bananas are the exception, having a glycemic load of 12.

Many years ago I introduced seven simple rules for healthy eating. My goal was to provide a common sense approach to eating that could be followed without consulting a book, using a calculator, or checking a list. Dozens of "Diet Books" and hundreds of articles have appeared since I introduced the seven rules, but they have not caused me to change my approach to healthy eating. The seven simple rules have stood the test of time. If you follow them you will greatly enhance your chances of living a long life, free of disease and disability.

Rule 1: Keep Your Diet Colorful

Fruits and vegetables provide most of the color to any meal. (Artificial colors don't count!) They are higher in nutrients and lower in saturated fats and empty calories than nearly anything else we eat. Their glycemic load is the lowest among carbohydrates and they are rich sources of fiber. They are an important part of what is referred to as a Mediterranean diet, which is now accepted by many authorities as one of the most healthy possible.

It is currently estimated that eating at least five servings of fruits and vegetables daily could reduce deaths from stroke, heart disease, and cancer by at least 20 percent. In light of this, it has been said that increasing consumption of fruits and vegetables ranks second only to smoking cessation as a means to prevent cancer.

One study showed that each portion of a fruit or vegetable eaten lowered the risk of heart attack by 4 percent and the risk of stroke by 6 percent. Other health benefits conveyed by fruits and vegetables include a lower risk of cataract development, an easing of asthma symptoms, improved bowel function, and improved control of diabetes.

Rule 2: Stick to Foods That Would Be Edible at Room Temperature

Foods that are high in saturated animal fat are unappealing at room temperature because the fat they contain has solidified. This gives them an unpleasing appearance and greasy taste. Studies continue to demonstrate that diets low in saturated fat convey health benefits, including longevity and a lower incidence of degenerative disease. *The China Study* by T. Colin Campbell, Ph.D., was released in 2004.[9] The book draws insights from dietary surveys done in China, where widely diverse patterns of disease are seen. The study's main conclusion is that diets containing a high percentage of animal fat and animal protein are one of the leading causes of cancer.

Rule 3: Avoid Refined Foods, Additives, and Preservatives

Refined sugars, flours, and grains carry very high glycemic loads. They are largely responsible for the dramatic rise in the incidence of Type 2 diabetes in the United States. Even children are being affected, as one in every three newly diagnosed childhood diabetics in Oklahoma has Type 2 diabetes. In addition, refined foods deplete B vitamin stores and adversely affect the body's immune system.

Rule 4: Include Oils That Are Liquid at Room Temperature

Evidence that oils from fatty, cold-water fish and plant oils such as olive oil, flaxseed oil, and evening primrose oil are essential to health continues to mount. Omega-3 fish oils, for example, have been reported to improve cholesterol ratios, prevent platelets from clumping together unnecessarily, improve mental function in children, and decrease the risk of heart irregularities and sudden death. These oils provide the building blocks the body needs to manufacture anti-inflammatory compounds, making them an effective tool in the management of arthritis and other inflammatory conditions.

Rule 5: Include Legumes (Beans and Peas)

It is no accident that beans were a staple of the frontier diet. They are low in cost, can easily be stored for long periods of time, and they provide a significant amount of high-quality protein and large amounts of fiber. Data demonstrating that ongoing consumption of legumes provides protection against heart disease and cancer continue to mount.

Soy is a legume that has both advocates and detractors. Substantial evidence suggests that regular consumption of soy foods lowers the risk of breast cancer, prostate cancer, and osteoporosis. Soy intake also lessens symptoms commonly associated with menopause.

In recent years, however, soy foods have been disparaged by some critics. Opponents of soy, some of whom attack its use as a food with evangelistic zeal, commonly set forth two arguments against its inclusion in a healthy diet. The first is that, due to the presence of substances that have an estrogen-like effect, soy consumption sends girls into early puberty and emasculates boys. The medical literature does not bear out these accusations. For over sixty years milk intolerant babies have been fed soy formulas. Long-term follow-up studies of infants raised exclusively on soy formula have shown no differences in onset of puberty, sexual characteristics, or fertility when compared to infants raised on milk-based formulas.

A second accusation is that soy consumption destroys thyroid activity. Evidence to support this allegation is meager, to say the least. It appears to be based upon a finding that a dosage adjustment is often required when infants receiving thyroid hormone replacement are changed from a cow's milk formula to a soy formula. No evidence exists to support the theory that a child or adult with normal thyroid function will be adversely affected by consuming soy products as part of a balanced diet.

A criticism that has merit suggests that many of today's soybean crops are being grown from genetically modified seed. This is true, but the same could be said of corn, tomatoes, and many other plant food sources. Non-GMO soy products are available, and I believe they should be chosen over soy products that are not labeled as being free of genetic modification.

Rule 6: Keep Meat Portions Small

The benefits of soy consumption may, in part, be due to a corresponding decrease in the consumption of meat and poultry. The China Study confirmed the findings of other studies showing that the consumption of meat and poultry (animal fat and animal protein) is associated with an increased risk of cancer development. As previously explained, animal protein, when metabolized, leaves an acidic ash that must be neutralized. If the amount of acid-producing food is too great for the body to neutralize effectively, body tissues will become acidic, a state that promotes cancer growth.

I strongly recommend that beef, pork, and poultry be viewed as condiments—items that are used in small amounts to add texture and flavor—rather than as the main course. Think of a "stir-fry" dish as an example. Stir-fry recipes call for relatively large amounts of vegetables flavored by a small amount of meat or seafood.

Rule 7: Vary What You Eat

Meals in the United States are usually very predictable: meat, potatoes, bread, and possibly a vegetable. Examples abound: A hamburger and fries (supersize that). Chicken salad and chips. A sirloin steak, a roll, and a baked-potato. When the diet is limited, so are the number of nutrients available from it. Increasing the number and types of foods consumed significantly increases the chance of obtaining needed nutrients.

Varying the diet also minimizes the chance of developing a food allergy or intolerance. Food allergies, which are quite common in our society, are almost always to foods that are being eaten more than twice a week. That most food allergies resolve if the offending food is avoided for three to six months and then eaten only at intervals of four or more days is well documented.

Whenever diet is discussed, the question of weight loss inevitably arises. I am confident that anyone who consistently follows the seven rules for healthy eating will experience as great or greater long-term success in weight control than that achieved by any "weight loss" regimen. Evidence strongly suggests that one's ideal weight is that reached by consistently maintaining habits that promote general wellness. Roller-coaster dieting is not only unsuccessful in achieving the goal of sustained weight loss, but it is also associated with higher risks of disease and premature death as well.

I strongly encourage you to stop pursuing the magical formula for weight loss and begin consistently following simple rules for healthy eating. Your ability to remain well throughout your lifetime depends upon it.

Remain Physically Active

Rosalie's aunt, Helen, needed exercise badly. There was only one problem . . . she *couldn't* exercise. There were many reasons. She was overweight. She had diabetes. She had arthritis. She had high blood pressure. She couldn't afford exercise equipment. She was housebound. One day Rosalie called her and suggested an activity. She might be able to set two soup cans by her recliner. Then she could periodically pick up one in each hand and move her arms back and forth as she watched TV.

Helen thought it sounded like a pretty good idea. She didn't have money to buy weights, but she could afford to set aside two cans of beans. She began "walking" with her arms for short periods of time. Within a few months she was walking a block to the post office in her small town. The postmaster installed a bench out front so that she could rest up for the trip home.

Before long Helen was walking around the block. Not exactly a marathon, but a tremendous step forward for an individual who had previously been unable to even get out in her own yard on a regular basis. The improvement in her quality of life was priceless.

While the words "exercise" and "activity" are to a large degree interchangeable, our emotional response to them is often much different. Helen benefited when she learned something that each of us should know. Even though we can't or don't want to exercise, we can and should be active. No one is beyond the point of being able to profit from an increased level of activity. We begin our lives as natural-born exercise addicts. If the infant or toddler is not sleeping, he or she is in constant motion. Arms are being waved and legs kicked, making diaper changes challenging. Unfortunately, we seem to lose our enthusiasm for exercise as we age. Many a grandparent has become worn out trying to keep up with a two- or three-year-old grandchild. This should not be the case, for we know that those who remain physically active are the most likely to enjoy health and vitality in their latter years.

It has often been said that the benefits of exercise are so great that if it could be bottled and sold as an elixir it would bring a fortune. A partial listing of these would include greater muscle strength and endurance, enhanced energy levels, improved mood, stronger bones, lower blood pressure, better balance, a lower percentage of body fat giving one a more striking appearance, and greater alertness. People who are physically fit are at significantly lower risk for disease or death than their non-fit peers. This is true even if individuals are "overweight" by conventional standards.

Three types of activities should be considered. These are aerobic activities, strengthening activities, and balance exercises. Aerobic activities are those that are done at an intensity that does not exceed the body's ability to supply oxygen to the muscles. Walking, jogging, cycling, swimming, and dance are examples of activities that can provide aerobic exercise.

Formulas have been devised to guide people toward the optimum level of aerobic activity. The most common is to exercise at 65 – 75 percent of one's maximum heart rate, determined by subtracting one's age from 220. For example, a forty–year-old would have a maximal heart rate of 220 – 40, or 180. Sixty-five percent of this would be 117 and 75 percent would be 135. Therefore, the target heart rate would be between 117 and 135. As fitness improves, an individual may be able to perform at 85 percent of the maximum heart rate. For a forty-year-old this would be 153. A simplified formula that works for most people is to gradually build up to a minimum heart rate of 120 and a maximum heart rate of 200 minus one's age. Using this formula, a forty-year-old's exercise pulse range would be from 120 to 160 beats per minute.

I dislike taking my pulse while walking and am not fond of formulas and calculations, however. I simply listen to what my body is telling me, walking at a pace that I find causes me to increase my breathing and break a light sweat, but at which I can still carry on a conversation or count out loud to ten periodically. An aerobic pace is one that an individual should be able to maintain for thirty minutes without difficulty, and at which he or she does not feel stiff the next day like a rusty tin man or woman who was left out in the rain.

Aerobic activities should be performed for twenty to thirty minutes three to five times each week. Strength training should also be done two to three times weekly. Weight lifting, resistance machines, push-ups, sit-ups, and similar exercises are common examples of strength training activities, but making beds and pushing a vacuum, or raking leaves, hoeing a garden, and cutting limbs are also strength building activities.

A regimen in which aerobic activities and strength training activities are done on alternate days is ideal for most people. Time constraints may prevent this, however. Busy people may choose to combine these two aspects of exercise. Increasing the number of repetitions and moving smoothly from one strengthening exercise to the next can result in an aerobic workout while doing strength training.

The third category of activities that should be performed regularly is balance exercises. These can be as simple as balancing on one foot for a minute then balancing on the other. If one is unable to stand on one foot, place the feet as close together as possible and attempt to maintain balance. Done regularly, activities of this type can markedly reduce the risk of falling and sustaining an injury.

While more exercise is better, even a little activity is good. Incorporating simple activities such as parking well away from a building rather than next to the door, taking the stairs rather than the elevator, and making your bed each morning will add to your well-being and decrease your risk of illness.

One bit of good news about exercise or activity is that it is never too late to start. Another is that benefits are often seen in a short period of time. The keys are to identify a starting point that is right for you, determine what activities you most enjoy and are willing to perform on a long-term consistent basis, and establish a time to do them that best fits your schedule.

Perhaps I should point out that while it is never too late to start an activity program, it is also never too early to begin. Any time is a great time to make a commitment to integrate regular physical activity into your routine. It is far easier to maintain the strength, endurance, and balance you currently possess than to recover it once it has been lost. You may be thinking, "That makes sense. I'm going to get started on an exercise regimen someday." You will never have a better opportunity to begin than you have today. Don't make the mistake of waiting for someday to arrive. It never will.

Treating your body like a palace by breathing clean air, drinking pure restored water, following the seven rules for healthy eating, and remaining physically active will provide a sound basis upon which to build health and longevity. If you go no further in your quest for optimum health you should do well, but the other measures revealed in this book will take you to progressively higher levels of protection against disease, disability, and premature death.

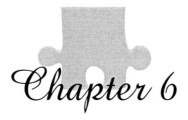

Chapter 6

Hire Bodyguards to Protect Your Cells from the Bullies

Is this not the fast that I have chosen: To loose the bonds of wickedness, To undo the heavy burdens, To let the oppressed go free, And that you break every yoke? Is it not to share your bread with the hungry, And that you bring to your house the poor who are cast out; When you see the naked, that you cover him, And not hide yourself from your own flesh? Then your light shall break forth like the morning, Your healing shall spring forth speedily, And your righteousness shall go before you; The glory of the LORD shall be your rear guard.
— Isaiah 58:6-8

One of the defining moments of my medical career took place at a most unusual location—the Frontier City Amusement Park in Oklahoma City. I had been bribed into attending a Saturday morning lecture at the park by a drug pusher, referred to in medical circles as a pharmaceutical representative. He had come to my office earlier that week and observed that one of my daughters was working in the reception area. He astutely pulled her aside and whispered, "If you can get your father to come to my program on Saturday morning, your whole family will be able to spend the whole day at the park for free!"

So there I was, listening to the umpteenth talk about cholesterol so the family could spend the rest of the day taking in the shows and enjoying the rides. I wasn't interested in what the speaker was saying; I had heard the same information many times before. To my amazement, he said something in the middle of his talk that caught my ear. I don't know if it caught the attention of any of the other physicians in attendance, but it certainly didn't register with the speaker himself since he went on to recommend the sponsor's cholesterol-lowering drug.

What captured my attention was this statement: LDL cholesterol, the so-called "bad" cholesterol, is harmless in its native state. Only when an LDL cholesterol molecule is attacked by a free radical and oxidized does it become subject to being pulled into the walls of an artery by a specialized white blood cell called a macrophage. Macrophage literally means "big eater." When a macrophage engulfs an oxidized LDL cholesterol molecule to pull it out of circulation and into the wall of an artery, it becomes a "foam cell," which is the first stage of an atherosclerotic plaque.

A light bulb lit up above my head, like a cartoon character that has an idea. "That means," I mused, "if I can figure out how to stop my LDL cholesterol from being oxidized, I won't have to follow in my father's footsteps and die of a heart attack in my early fifties." I had just been introduced to free radical damage, one of the mechanisms of disease and aging. This lecture unexpectedly changed my medical perspective and dramatically altered the direction of my life!

Understanding Free Radicals

In order to understand what free radicals are and how they accelerate disease development and aging, it is necessary to review basic chemistry. All matter, including the human body, is composed of atoms. Atoms are made up of positively charged protons, negatively charged electrons, and uncharged particles called neutrons. Protons and neutrons are found in the nucleus of the atom and electrons are found in shells surrounding the nucleus.

An atom will be either stable or unstable depending upon the number of electrons in its outer shell. The first shell of an atom is stable when two electrons are present. The other shells become stable when eight electrons are present. The most stable elements are called noble gases, which include helium, neon, and others. Helium is stable because it has two electrons in its only shell. All other noble gases are stable because they have eight electrons in their outer shell.

Atoms that do not have a stable number of electrons in their outer shell can become stable by partnering with another atom that is similarly unstable. Balance can be achieved in two ways. It can be accomplished by sharing electrons, a process called covalent bonding, or by one atom donating one or more electrons to an atom that needs one or more electrons. Ionic bonding is the name given to the donating and receiving process. Stable molecules consist of atoms that have become balanced through covalent or ionic bonding.

A free radical is an atom or molecule with unpaired electrons in its outer shell. Because they are unbalanced, free radicals are highly reactive. This is not necessarily a bad thing. Free radicals can be extremely useful under the proper circumstances. In the environment, oxygen free radicals are useful in producing energy through such methods as burning wood in a fireplace or gasoline in an internal combustion engine. Free radicals are necessary for metabolism (energy production) in our body. Some free radicals help to control the tone of our arteries and others are important tools of our body's immune system.

Free radicals are necessary for energy production, but they can cause a great deal of damage as well. In the environment, free radicals cause metals to rust, pictures and window treatments to fade, fats to turn rancid, tires to dry rot, and car finishes to fade. When a car finish has faded in the sun, it is said to have oxidized. In the body, free radicals attack cell membranes, DNA, and molecules such as LDL cholesterol. When an LDL cholesterol molecule has been attacked by a free radical and changed in appearance, it is said to have oxidized, just as in the case of a faded car finish.

Free radicals that play a significant role in aging and disease development are unbalanced molecules that contain oxygen. These are called oxygen free radicals and they come from many sources. Some oxygen free radicals are formed as ultraviolet light displaces electrons in oxygen molecules as sunlight passes through the atmosphere. Other free radicals form in the human body during periods of physical exercise and when an individual is under emotional stress. They're a natural byproduct of cellular energy production, and they are generated as molecules are exposed to heat or enzymatic activity. They are also created when the body is exposed to radiation or chemotherapy. Free radicals are also found in smog and cigarette smoke. (A single puff of cigarette smoke contains approximately one quadrillion [1,000,000,000,000,000] free radicals.)[10]

Significant Free Radicals

Several free radicals are of major significance to the human body. These are superoxide, the hydroxyl radical, hydrogen peroxide, and the lipid peroxyl radical. Although it is technically not a free radical, singlet oxygen behaves in a similar manner and so it will be included in the discussion. Now let's define those terms and give you an idea of how they behave in the body.

Superoxide is called the "master oxygen radical" because it leads to the formation of many other free radicals. It is the mob boss of the free radical world. Superoxide is formed when a free electron attaches to an oxygen molecule. Since the oxygen molecule now has an extra electron it is no longer stable. Superoxide easily converts to hydrogen peroxide or the hydroxyl radical.

The hydroxyl radical is the most damaging free radical in the body. I am sure that the chemical formula of water, H_2O, is familiar to you. Because water is made up of two hydrogen atoms and one oxygen atom, it is balanced and very stable. On the other hand, the hydroxyl radical has only one hydrogen atom, which only partially balances the oxygen atom. As a result, the hydroxyl radical attacks nearly any molecule with which it comes into contact. Its aggressiveness can be appreciated through the fact that the average length of time a hydroxyl radical exists before partnering with another molecule is 0.000000001 second. The hydroxyl radical is the mafia hit man in the body.

Hydrogen peroxide is commonly used for its bleaching properties. Hydrogen peroxide is reactive because it has two hydrogen atoms paired with two oxygen atoms. This means that the compound must acquire two additional electrons to become stable. One of the dangerous characteristics of hydrogen peroxide is its ability to pass through cell membranes and damage the interior of cells. Think of hydrogen peroxide as a home invader.

Hydrogen peroxide reacts with superoxide or iron to form the hydroxyl radical. This has caused some health practitioners to brand iron a dangerous element in spite of the fact that red blood cells cannot be manufactured if iron levels are insufficient. Iron should not be feared if the body's antioxidant defenses are working properly.

The lipid peroxyl radical is a wolf that comes disguised in sheep's clothing. It is formed in two ways. It is left behind when the body burns animal fat, and it is also formed when oxygen free radicals attack fats that are found in cell membranes. The formation of the lipid peroxyl radical triggers a chain reaction creating additional free radicals across the cell membrane. This can result in damage to important cell components including DNA. DNA damage is one of the primary triggers of cancer development.

Singlet oxygen is like a ninja sniper. It is formed mainly in the skin in response to ultraviolet light. Singlet oxygen has the same chemical formula of stable oxygen, O_2, but its shared electrons are spinning in opposite directions.

This causes instability. Singlet oxygen's existence is extremely short as it immediately attacks other substances to achieve balance. Singlet oxygen is believed to contribute to the development of skin cancer.

The Body's Antioxidant Defenses

The body's antioxidant defense mechanism is designed to deal with free radicals before DNA, LDL cholesterol, cell membranes, or other substances are damaged. By using its antioxidant defenses, the body is able to increase the stabilization process of free radicals by a factor of ten million. This means that free radicals should be neutralized before they do any harm. As long as the body's defenses are able to keep up with free radical exposure all is well; damage occurs when the body's defenses are outnumbered by free radicals and become overwhelmed.

I often see articles recommending the use of vitamin E and vitamin C as antioxidants. Some may add selenium. This is overly simplistic. Medical studies looking at the supplementation of a single nutrient such as vitamin E or beta carotene have demonstrated that the outcome is actually worse with supplementation than without. This has led people to believe that nutritional supplementation, specifically antioxidant supplementation, is harmful or dangerous. This is an incorrect interpretation of the study findings. Actually, supporting the body's antioxidant defense system is appropriate and necessary, provided that support is comprehensive. The body's antioxidant defense system needs privates and lieutenants as well as colonels and generals.

The outcome of single nutrient studies should have been anticipated in advance for they provide an incomplete solution. When vitamin E, for example, donates an electron to disarm and balance a free radical, vitamin E itself becomes unbalanced. Unless it is quickly rebalanced, it will act as any other free radical and attack surrounding molecules. This is a challenge because, being fat soluble, vitamin E will remain in the body for extended periods of time. Vitamin C, on the other hand, is water soluble and therefore washes out of the body very quickly. In the short time it is in the body, however, vitamin C works to balance and neutralize free radicals. It is even capable of recycling the wounded vitamin E so vitamin E can return to the front lines as an antioxidant rather than as a free radical. Supplementing vitamin E without providing a means for it to be recycled has the potential to do more harm than good, as the single nutrient studies have shown. As in the case of vitamin C and vitamin E, multiple antioxidant defenders are needed to watch each other's backs.

If an adequate supply of raw materials is available, the body will manufacture a number of antioxidants. Several of these are enzymes, substances that drive chemical reactions without reacting with the other substances involved. In other words, enzymes are facilitators. Antioxidant enzymes include superoxide dismutase, glutathione peroxidase, and catalase. These are long names, but we need to know something about them to fully appreciate the incredibly effective design of the body's antioxidant army.

Superoxide dismutase protects against the mob boss, the superoxide radical. It does this by driving the chemical reaction that changes the superoxide radical to hydrogen peroxide. The job is not finished, but in so doing it blocks the production of the most damaging hydroxyl radical. The reaction requires mineral cofactors including manganese, zinc, and copper, so deficiencies in these elements will prevent superoxide dismutase from performing its protective assignment effectively. The need for these minerals is an example of why providing comprehensive nutritional support is so important.

Glutathione peroxidase completes what superoxide dismutase started by donating an electron to neutralize hydrogen peroxide. This also blocks the production of the dreaded hydroxyl radical. Glutathione peroxidase is then recycled by another enzyme, glutathione reductase. Production of the glutathione enzymes requires the availability of amino acids and selenium, which are also found in high quality comprehensive supports.

Catalase converts bullying hydrogen peroxide to friendly water and oxygen. That process is dependent upon the availability of iron. (This is further evidence that the claim that iron intake should be restricted is short-sighted and not based upon a complete understanding of body function.)

In addition to enzymes, the body manufactures substances called quencher molecules and uses them to limit free radical damage. One quencher is uric acid, which protects against several bullies including superoxide, hydroxyl, and lipid peroxyl radicals. Uric acid is as effective as vitamin C in this process. Another is ceruloplasmin that protects against superoxide, the hydroxyl radical, and singlet oxygen.

Thus, it is clear that a diverse team of bodyguards is required to protect the body from free radical bullies. While the popular antioxidant nutrients vitamin

E and vitamin C are important in stopping oxidation in the body, many other nutrients must be provided if the body's antioxidant defenses are to be successful. Vitamin A neutralizes singlet oxygen and lipid peroxyl radicals. Vitamin C neutralizes superoxide and hydroxyl radicals. It also recycles vitamin E. Vitamin E neutralizes singlet oxygen and lipid peroxyl radicals. B vitamins are needed to regenerate glutathione peroxidase. The importance of the minerals selenium, zinc, copper, and iron has been explained above.

The Role of Bioflavanoids

Bioflavanoids are plant-based compounds that directly scavenge free radicals in addition to enhancing the activity of vitamin C and vitamin E. Over five hundred bioflavanoids are known including oligoproanthocyanidins (don't try to pronounce that; just call them OPCs). These "good guys" include grape seed and pine bark extracts, tannins from teas, anthocyanins from dark fruits, and silymarin from milk thistle.

Since virtually all fruits contain bioflavanoids, it has become common for companies to search out fruits with exotic names to obtain a competitive edge in the antioxidant marketplace. Fifteen years ago, almost no one in the United States was aware of the existence of fruits such as noni, gogi, mangosteen, or acai. Thanks to the aggressive marketing, many Americans are drinking juice mixtures that contain at least one exotic fruit. It is true that the exotics provide strong antioxidant benefit, but it is difficult to show that they are superior to common (and much less expensive) juices such as grape, cranberry, or cherry.

A key characteristic of bioflavanoids is their ability to cross what is called the blood-brain barrier. The blood-brain barrier is a mechanism that prevents entry of potentially toxic substances into the sensitive central nervous system including the brain and spinal cord. While the blood-brain barrier plays a key role in protecting the brain from toxins, it can also leave the brain susceptible to free radical damage by blocking entry of vitamin C and vitamin E.

In the late 1990s, I attended a symposium on two degenerative conditions of the brain, Alzheimer's Disease and Parkinson's Disease. One of the nation's leading researchers in diseases of the central nervous system stated that if a way was ever discovered to get vitamin C into the brain it would represent a giant leap forward in the prevention of those debilitating diseases. The good news is that we do know how to get vitamin C into the brain. OPCs like grape seed extract freely cross the blood-brain barrier and when they do they carry vitamin C and vitamin E with them. Sadly, conventional American medicine is not open to the use of plant extracts in preventing major illness; it is willing to look only to the pharmaceutical industry for answers to health challenges.

Other antioxidant nutrients include coenzyme Q10 and N-acetyl cysteine. Coenzyme Q10 is particularly beneficial in low oxygen states, such as congestive heart failure or emphysema. N-acetyl cysteine, while exhibiting antioxidant properties of its own, also enhances the production of glutathione, which is needed in the manufacturing of the very important enzyme, glutathione peroxidase.

Stopping oxidative damage from free radicals is one of the secrets to a long and healthy life. Specific steps that can be taken to lessen oxidative damage include minimizing time spent in smoggy environments, avoiding cigarette smoke, eating a diet rich in fruits and vegetables, and providing support to the body's antioxidant defense system through nutritional bodyguards. I have explained why antioxidant supplementation must not be limited to two or three key nutrients. It should include a balanced support product that contains all of the vitamins, minerals, and amino acids needed to produce antioxidant substances, along with an OPC such as grape seed extract. Coenzyme Q10 should be added when low-oxygen conditions are present.

Successfully protecting one's body from free radical damage need not be complicated or costly. The simple steps detailed above will tip the battle in the body's favor and add productive years to your life.

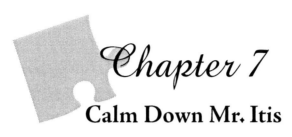

Chapter 7

Calm Down Mr. Itis

Do not be wise in your own eyes; Fear the LORD and depart from evil.
It will be health to your flesh, And strength to your bones.
– Proverbs 3:7-8

"What prompted you to come and see me today?" I asked the elderly gentleman seated next to my desk in the examination room.

"Arthur is paying me a visit," he responded. I immediately knew what was to come next (I've heard the joke many times over the years), but I played along.

"Arthur who?" I asked.

"Arthur Itis!" he snapped, letting out a hearty laugh. His mood quickly turned somber, however. "It's really not a laughing matter," he confessed. "It's come to the point where my joints never stop hurting. Is there anything that can give me some relief?"

He was not alone in his plight. It is said that over half of people over the age of sixty-five live in constant pain. This is usually due to arthritis or one of the many other conditions that are characterized by chronic inflammation. Mr. Itis comes in many forms—bursitis, cystitis, tendonitis, hepatitis, and gastritis are just a few of his aliases. The suffix "itis" means inflammation and its attachment to any body part means that tissue or organ is inflamed.

Acute and Chronic Inflammation

Inflammation is not meant to be harmful. It is, in fact, one of the body's primary healing mechanisms. Inflammation is the body's basic response to a variety of external or internal insults, such as infectious agents, physical injury, hypoxia (low oxygen levels), or disease processes in nearly any organ or tissue in the body. Signs of inflammation include redness, heat, tenderness or pain, and swelling.

Examples of acute inflammation include a burn, an insect bite, frostbite, and the fever and aching accompanying a flu-like illness. Acute inflammation can promote healing; chronic inflammation can lead to a wide range of disease states and significantly accelerate the aging process.

Some of the conditions that are triggered or aggravated by chronic inflammation are allergies, Alzheimer's disease, anemia, arthritis, atherosclerosis, cancer, collagen diseases (rheumatoid arthritis, systemic lupus erythematosis, scleroderma, and dermatomyositis), congestive heart failure, Crohn's disease, ulcerative colitis, fibromyalgia, Hashimoto's thyroiditis, kidney failure, multiple sclerosis, and psoriasis. Any condition that ends in "itis" has an inflammatory cause. Calming down chronic inflammation can easily add a decade or more to a person's life span. More importantly, keeping it under control can help assure that those extra years are characterized not by pain, but by activity.

The degree to which chronic inflammation affects longevity can be appreciated by considering that inflammation is the initial event that leads to the development of the two greatest killers in our society—atherosclerosis (hardening of the arteries) and cancer. Inflammatory injury to the lining of arteries creates the condition necessary for deposition of plaque in arteries. In November 2005 a Japanese researcher, Dr. H. Okuyama, reported that supplementation of omega-3 oils is more effective in preventing heart attacks than use of cholesterol-lowering medications.[11] Some are now proposing that popular statin drugs reduce heart attack risk not by lowering cholesterol, but by producing a separate anti-inflammatory effect. Nearly all cancers begin with inflammation. A severe sunburn triggers the development of skin cancer, inflammation caused by a papilloma virus infection leads to cervical cancer, inflammation of the mouth, bronchial tubes, and esophagus caused by cigarette smoke predisposes to cancers in those areas, and chronic inflammation in the prostate creates an environment that leads to prostate cancer. It is therefore imperative that steps be taken to identify and reverse chronic inflammation when it is present.

Markers of Inflammation

A number of chemical markers of inflammation exist, which can be monitored by blood tests. One of the simplest tests for inflammation is the erythrocyte sedimentation rate (ESR). The ESR indicates that proteins from an inflammatory process are in the bloodstream and are causing red blood cells to stick together. The ESR test is quite simple to do. Blood is drawn into a small tube. The tube is placed upright and after an hour the distance that the red blood cells have fallen is measured in millimeters. Since clumps of red blood cells are heavier and fall more quickly than individual red blood cells, the rate of settling rises as the amount of inflammation present in the body increases.

Sedimentation rates up to 15 mm/hr in men and 20 mm/hr in women under the age of fifty are considered normal. After the age of fifty, the upper limit of normal is considered to be 20 mm/hr in men and 30 mm/hr in women. It is important to note that these values are "normal" only in that typically no identifiable disease process is present in that range; "normal" values do not mean that no inflammation is present. The higher levels seen in people over fifty are in all likelihood due to inflammatory processes that have not yet progressed far enough for a disease to be recognized.

C-reactive protein (CRP) is a protein that is manufactured in the liver and in fat cells. Low amounts are always present, but levels can rise dramatically when inflammation is present. CRP is considered an acute phase reactant, meaning that it is an important factor in the body's immediate response to infection. CRP helps the body mark foreign substances for removal by white blood cells. It also enhances the ability of white blood cells to engulf and destroy bacteria, viruses, and foreign proteins.

It has been found that higher than usual baseline levels of CRP are associated with an increased risk for heart attack. Individuals who have a baseline level of CRP less than 1 mg/L are considered to be at low risk for heart disease, those with levels between 1 and 3 are felt to be at average risk, and people with CRP levels above 3 when no infection is present are said to be at high risk for a future heart attack.

C-reactive protein production is closely linked to a substance called interleukin-6 (IL-6). IL-6 is a member of a family of chemicals called cytokines. Cytokines are responsible for intercellular communication in the body. Interleukin-6 can play an anti-inflammatory role at times. IL-6 is released with muscle activity and stimulates burning of fat and improved usage of insulin. When an infection occurs, white blood cells manufacture IL-6. The increasing amounts of IL-6 in an infection trigger increased production of C-reactive protein in the liver.

Other inflammatory cytokines that can be measured to monitor inflammation in the body include tumor necrosis factor alpha (TNF-a), interleukin-1 beta (IL-1b), and interleukin-8 (IL-8). Low levels of cholesterol also suggest that inflammation is present. None of the inflammatory markers tell where the inflammation is or what is causing it. They simply give an indication of the degree of inflammation that is present in the body at any point in time.

Causes of Chronic Inflammation

Many underlying causes of chronic inflammation have been identified, and most can be addressed successfully. One of the factors responsible for chronic inflammation is lack of adequate sleep. When sleep is insufficient, levels of IL-6 have been found to increase by 40 – 60 percent and levels of TNF-a by 20 – 30 percent. C-reactive protein levels rise accordingly.

Chronic stress often leads to adrenal fatigue, a condition in which the adrenal glands are unable to keep up with the body's demand for adrenaline, noradrenaline, and cortisol. Since cortisol is one of the body's primary anti-inflammatory substances, adrenal fatigue results in chronic inflammation. How stress is handled is critically important, as emotions play a role in creating chronic inflammation. For example, CRP has been shown to increase in response to anger, hostility, or depressive feelings.

Since IL-6 and CRP are both manufactured in fat cells, obesity is often characterized by chronic inflammation. This is true in young people as well as older individuals. The role of chronic inflammation in the development of cancer and diseases of the circulatory system explains, at least in part, why obesity carries a higher risk for development of chronic disease and premature death.

Diet plays a major role in determining the amount of inflammation in the body. My father-in-law, a Minnesota dairy farmer, was a man that occasionally enjoyed a little bread with his butter. No meal setting was complete without a generous supply of the smooth, yellow spread. The introduction of oleomargarine upset him greatly.

His dislike of margarine was not based solely upon the potential economic effect on his business. He saw this interloper, cosmetically designed to have a texture and appearance similar to his beloved spread, as a threat to the long-term health and well being of those who chose to consume it. It can't be good for you, he insisted, it's not a real food.

Time has proven that his assessment was correct. Hydrogenated fats and trans fatty acids, the chemically altered substances that give margarine the appearance and texture of butter, are now recognized as significant factors in the atherogenic process—the "hardening of the arteries" that leads to heart attacks, strokes, and other serious threats to health. The latter half of the twentieth century will almost certainly be viewed historically as the era during which the human race, believing that it could eliminate disease by improving upon the foods that had been provided to it, discovered how to effectively create epidemics of diabetes, obesity, atherosclerosis, cancer, ADHD, and a host of other chronic and often fatal illnesses.

Despite eating diets high in overall fat content, surveys have shown that most people in the United States are obtaining only ten percent of the fats they need to maintain optimum health. The fats the body requires for effective maintenance and repair functions are called essential fatty acids (EFAs). The term "essential" means that we are incapable of manufacturing these substances and must obtain them from our diet. Several factors account for the widespread essential fatty acid deficiencies seen today.

The first is the modification of naturally occurring fats. Essential fatty acids are found in mono and polyunsaturated fats. Because these fats are liquid at room temperature, they do not work well as butter substitutes or as ingredients in packaged foods. Adding additional chemical entities to unsaturated fats causes them to become solid at room temperature, making them more acceptable as spreads or as additions to packaged foods.

Unfortunately, these modified fats called "hydrogenated" or "trans" fats cannot be utilized by the body. In addition, they have been shown to play a significant role in the development of atherosclerosis.

The second factor contributing to fatty acid deficiencies is an imbalance of the types of essential fatty acids in the diet. Two categories of essential fatty acids exist. These are referred to as omega-6 and omega-3 fatty acids.

Because corn and other vegetable oil products most commonly sold in grocery stores and the oils most commonly added to processed foods, are high in omega-6 fatty acids, most people obtain more than enough omega-6 fatty acids from the foods they eat. Very few, however, obtain significant quantities of omega-3 oils from their diet. While a 4:1 ratio of omega-6 to omega-3 oils is considered optimum, most Americans consume more than 20 times more omega-6 oils than omega-3 oils on a daily basis. To understand how this impacts our health, it is necessary to know something about a group of substances called prostaglandins.

The Role of Prostaglandins

In the 1930s, a Swedish scientist, Ulf von Euler, identified a new chemical in fluid from the prostate gland. He named the chemical prostaglandin. We now know that such chemicals are not unique to the prostate, but are manufactured throughout the body to produce a wide variety of effects. Unlike hormones, which are made in specialized glands and distributed throughout the body, prostaglandins are manufactured on location and act only in that location.

Prostaglandins influence a wide array of body reactions. They affect the amount of protective mucus lining the stomach, trigger the onset of labor, and can cause constriction in bronchial tubes. Some prostaglandins trigger inflammation while others fight inflammation. Certain prostaglandins encourage the formation of blood clots; others keep the blood from clotting.

While the medical community commonly speaks of "good" prostaglandins and "bad" prostaglandins, such labels are misleading. Prostaglandins simply do what they are manufactured to do. Whether the end result of their action is beneficial or harmful is not determined by the presence of "good" or "bad" prostaglandins, but by the body's ability to manufacture the proper prostaglandin in any particular situation.

Viewing prostaglandins as "bad" can lead to undesirable complications. I am very concerned about the challenge of iatrogenic illness—injury or death due to adverse effects of medical diagnostic procedures and treatments. NSAIDs, non-steroidal anti-inflammatory drugs, are a leading cause of iatrogenic disease. As the name implies, they are the standard medical treatment for conditions associated with inflammation.

NSAIDs work by blocking the body's ability to manufacture a substance called arachidonic acid, which leads to the production of inflammatory prostaglandins. Unfortunately, these drugs also block the body's ability to manufacture prostaglandins that are responsible for protecting the lining of the stomach from the caustic action of hydrochloric acid, compromise kidney function, and place people at risk for heart failure. This can have disastrous consequences, as demonstrated by a report, published in *the American Journal of Medicine*, that 16,500 people in the United States died in 1997 as a direct result of the use of these drugs.[12]

Fatty Acid Deficiencies

In nearly all instances, it is not necessary to accept the risks of NSAIDs. All that is required is to provide the body with ample amounts of omega-3 fatty acids and systemic enzymes.

Given an adequate supply of raw materials, the body will manufacture the proper prostaglandin in every situation. When deficiencies exist, however, the body's attempt to correct a challenge can result in the production of the wrong prostaglandin for the condition.

Imagine that an architect has designed a building that is to have a fascia composed of four red bricks for each black brick. This calls for sixteen loads of red bricks and four loads of black bricks. If the masons are supplied with 19 loads of red bricks and only one load of black bricks, they can still complete the building. Its appearance, however, will not be what the architect intended.

When an individual's diet contains 19 omega-6 fatty acids for each omega-3 fatty acid, the body cannot follow the blueprint it has been given. It will do its best, but the end result may not be what the Architect intended.

Platelets and blood clots are an excellent example. The blueprint for platelets calls for an alternating pattern of fats within their membranes. If the body does not have enough omega-3 fats to complete the platelet membrane as designed, it will use the fats it has on hand to complete the job. Improperly constituted platelet membranes, however, are "sticky" and tend to cause platelets to clump together.

Certain prostaglandins that are dependent upon the availability of omega-3 fatty acids for their manufacture decrease platelet stickiness and discourage clot formation. If the body does not have an adequate supply of omega-3 fats it will do its best, but the prostaglandins produced with omega-6 oils will increase platelet aggregation and stimulate clot formation.

The lack of omega-3 fats in the American diet forces the body to manufacture platelets that are sticky and prostaglandins that promote the formation of blood clots. The medical community has responded by recommending that people take an aspirin a day. Aspirin prevents platelets from sticking together in situations where a heart attack or stroke could occur, but it also prevents platelets from clumping and clots from forming when bleeding occurs. This increases the risk of bruising or bleeding when bumped or injured. It also significantly increases the risk of a bleed into the brain, an event known as a hemorrhagic stroke. A better approach is to allow the body to build platelets as the Architect intended and choose which prostaglandins should be manufactured by providing an ample supply of omega-3 fatty acids.

Omega-3 fatty acids are needed in the manufacturing of anti-inflammatory prostaglandins, while omega-6 fatty acids are used in the production of inflammatory compounds. Diets low in omega-3 fatty acids or having a high ratio of omega-6 to omega-3 oils, which are common in the United States, promote the production of inflammatory prostaglandins. Meats and dairy products are high in arachidonic acid, the primary omega-6 fatty acid required for the production of inflammatory prostaglandins. It should come as no surprise that people who eat a diet high in animal fat experience more inflammatory conditions than those who eat diets that are predominantly plant-based.

Asthma can be used to demonstrate how imbalances of dietary fat affect the presence and severity of disease. Inflammation is one of the root causes of asthma. Cortisone-like drugs have traditionally been used to calm inflammation in the bronchial tubes and reduce the frequency and severity of asthma attacks. More recently, drugs designed to inhibit the action of substances called leukotrienes have been introduced.

Leukotrienes are closely related to prostaglandins. Just as in the case of prostaglandins, the body can produce either inflammatory or anti-inflammatory leukotrienes, provided the proper balance of fatty acids is available. Inflammatory leukotrienes dominate when a high omega-6 to omega-3 fatty acid ratio is present.

When the diet is deficient in omega-3 fatty acids, leukotrienes and prostaglandins that cause bronchial tubes to narrow and constrict are produced.

Supplementation of omega-3 fatty acids can result in significant improvement in asthma by restoring the body's ability to manufacture prostaglandins that encourage relaxation and opening of the bronchial tubes and reduced production of inflammatory leukotrienes.

Systemic Enzymes – The Body's Clean-up Crew

Diets that consist primarily of cooked food also promote inflammation. They do so by depleting the body's supply of systemic enzymes and by promoting the attachment of glucose to protein.

I can best describe the role of systemic enzymes in the body by comparing it to a terrorist attack. On April 19, 1995, life in Oklahoma City changed forever. In an instant, the front half of the nine-story Murrah Federal Building was reduced to a pile of rubble. Ragged structural fragments dangled from sections of the building that remained standing. In the days that followed, I—like many in the area—drove to the site to view the damage firsthand. It is a scene I shall never forget.

A visit to the location today is quite different than in the days following the blast. The debris is gone. In its place stand empty chairs on a grassy hill overlooking a reflecting pond. It is a serene oasis in the midst of the city, a place where healing can take place.

The transition from chaos to beauty did not take place overnight, nor was it the result of chance. The transition was facilitated by clean-up crews that removed the rubble piece by piece until the site was clear and prepared for renovation. Without the work of the clean-up crews, restoration of the site could not have taken place.

The Murrah bombing and the more recent Trade Center attacks are examples of what is taking place within our bodies on an ongoing basis. As long as we are alive, the sequence of damage, clean-up, and restoration never ends. It is estimated that each of our cells is attacked by a free radical 10,000 times a day. It is also said that a cancer, a blood clot, and an arterial plaque begin to form every second of our lives. Injury is an unavoidable reality of life. Inflammatory debris appears whenever an injury occurs. Without clean-up crews, this debris would accumulate within the body and healing could not take place. Were it not for the presence of efficient clean-up crews within our bodies we would die in a relatively short period of time.

The body's clean-up workers are called enzymes. Technically, an enzyme is a substance that initiates a chemical reaction or enables the reaction to proceed more efficiently than would normally be the case. Enzymes are essential to nearly all body processes. Over 10,000 different enzymes have been identified and registered to date. They play a major role in the digestion of our food, break down toxic substances to facilitate their elimination from the body, aid in the building of new cells and tissues, and direct the conversion of stored fat and glycogen to useful energy.

Enzymatic action can be readily observed by placing a freshly picked piece of fruit on a kitchen counter and simply leaving it there. Within a few days, the fruit will begin to rot. This is the result of naturally occurring enzymes within the fruit digesting the pulp to release the seed inside. Enzymes are very sensitive to heat, however. If a piece of freshly picked fruit is heated before it is set on the counter, it will never rot. It may mold over time, but it will not decay, since the enzymes it contained have been destroyed.

Pancreatic enzymes support the digestive process by breaking down food as it passes through the intestinal tract. Pancreatic enzymes that are not required for food digestion circulate through the body looking for sites of debris and inflammation. When inflammation is encountered, the enzymes go to work clearing debris from the area so that healing can take place.

Raw foods contain enzymes that aid in their digestion, but cooked foods do not. When cooked food is eaten, the body must use more pancreatic enzymes in the digestive process than when food is eaten raw or lightly steamed. As a result there are fewer enzymes available to deal with inflammation throughout the body.

The other reason that diets high in cooked foods promote inflammation is that they increase the rate of glycosylation, which is the mechanism by which glucose is attached to proteins. Glycosylation accelerates the aging process by causing proteins to stiffen. A common test of blood sugar control in diabetes is called a glycosylated hemoglobin or A1C test. The test looks at the stiffness of red blood cells. The higher the blood sugar over time, the faster the glycosylation process progresses. Therefore, the degree to which red blood cells have stiffened is a reflection of the average blood sugar over the two- to three-month time frame preceding the test. Protein glycosylation triggers the release of inflammatory cytokines such as IL-6, leading to chronic inflammation.

Other Causes of Chronic Inflammation

Deficiencies of vitamin D and copper also predispose to the development of inflammatory conditions. As vitamin D levels fall, amounts of the inflammatory cytokine TNF alpha rise. Relatively small amounts of vitamin D in the 400 IU daily range have been shown to lower TNF-alpha levels. Copper is needed to help the body produce a proper balance of prostaglandins. This is at least a partial explanation of why the wearing of a copper bracelet will often improve arthritic symptoms.

Persistent, low-grade infections are another cause of chronic inflammation. Some of the entities that are capable of causing chronic infection are chlamydia pneumoniae, helicobacter pylori, herpes simplex, cytomegalovirus, and the human papilloma virus. If inflammatory markers such as C-reactive protein are found to be elevated, a careful search for the presence of chronic infections should be conducted.

Controlling Chronic Inflammation

Steps that can be taken to control chronic inflammation include reducing stress, maintaining a positive outlook, losing weight, eating a wellness diet, increasing the percentage of raw or lightly steamed foods in the diet, finding and addressing chronic infections, and providing nutritional supports. The two supports critical to control of chronic inflammation are omega-3 fatty acids and enzymes.

Omega-3 fatty acids provide the body with the raw materials required to shift production from inflammatory to non-inflammatory prostaglandins. Animal sources of omega-3 oils include cold water fish oils, krill oil, cod-liver oil, and green-lipped mussel oil. I find fish oils to be the most economical and recommend that enough be taken to provide 600 mg. of EPA (eicosapentaenoic acid) and 400 mg. of DHA (docosahexaenoic acid) daily. Plant-based sources include flaxseed oil, borage oil, evening primrose oil, walnut oil, and hemp oil. Of these, flaxseed oil is the most economical.

When using flaxseed oil it is important to recognize that the optimum amount is one to two tablespoons daily. I do not recommend flaxseed oil capsules for a very simple reason—the capsules do not provide nearly enough oil to obtain significant benefit. Fourteen capsules are required to provide one tablespoon of oil. Therefore, fourteen to twenty-eight flaxseed oil capsules must be taken to obtain an optimum daily serving, an amount that few would be willing to swallow on a daily basis.

As a physician, I was taught that enzymes could not be supplemented. Many physicians still believe that oral enzyme supplements cannot be used effectively. The thought is that the enzyme molecules will be broken down before being absorbed, making the supplements worthless. This has been shown to be incorrect. Enzymes are absorbed and go to work cleaning up debris and performing other tasks within the body when taken orally.

Much of the initial research of systemic enzymes was done in Europe. During the 1960s and 1970s, East German athletes dominated world competitions. East German sports scientists were highly advanced in creating training regimens. They were the first to use anabolic steroids for strength enhancement. This practice is now known to be dangerous and has been banned in nearly all sports.

While the East Germans' use of steroids received a great deal of coverage, one of their greatest advances, the use of safe and legal systemic enzymes, did not. It was not until the mid 1990s, long after the fall of the Berlin wall, that an East German official explained that a great deal of the country's athletic success had been due to the use of systemic enzymes, which they had purchased through middlemen in various European cities.

Without the use of systemic enzymes, the anabolic steroid administration would not have been successful. Each time an athlete trains, tendons, ligaments, and joints are traumatized to a degree. These daily microtraumas make the athlete more susceptible to major sprains, strains, and similar injuries.

The East German trainers discovered that relatively low quantities of systemic enzymes were capable of protecting athletes from the effects of microtrauma and that higher amounts could significantly shorten the amount of time needed for recovery from major injuries. In addition, they had found that the regular use of systemic enzymes during training enhanced muscle development, strength, and endurance.[13]

Hundreds of published studies have now documented the effectiveness of systemic enzymes in reducing inflammation, swelling, and internal bleeding associated with athletic injuries. A 1996 report on Ukrainian athletes typifies the results.[14] Thirty-one members of the Ukraine soccer and karate teams suffered severe sprains or strains. Half of them were given systemic enzyme supplements. The others received aggressive medical treatment including compresses, heparin, non-steroidal anti-inflammatory drugs, physical therapy, novocaine, and hydrocortisone.

The athletes given systemic enzymes reported significant pain relief within two days and returned to training three and a half weeks post injury. The group given medical treatment did not report pain relief for seven to nine days and did not resume training for six weeks. I have observed similar results in recommending systemic enzyme supplementation to people who have consulted me with injuries ranging from severe sprains to large contusions (bruises).

Systemic enzymes work so effectively in helping the body resolve injuries because they significantly reduce the associated inflammation. They "clean up the debris" so that optimum healing can take place. Their effectiveness in reducing inflammation makes them effective in a wide variety of situations.

Numerous studies have demonstrated that systemic enzymes work as effectively, often more effectively, than non-steroidal anti-inflammatory drugs in relieving the pain and inflammation associated with arthritis. Unlike NSAIDs, however, systemic enzymes are not associated with significant side effects, and no deaths have resulted from their use. While the *American Journal of Medicine* reported in 1997 that 16,500 people in the United States die each year from properly prescribed and administered NSAIDs, in 1992 the German Health Service reported 1.4 million prescriptions of systemic enzyme preparations without a single severe adverse effect.[15] Systemic enzymes effectively counter chronic inflammation as reflected by lower levels of C-reactive protein.[16]

Systemic enzymes must be taken on an empty stomach to be effective. They will go to work cleaning up the first debris they encounter, which, if taken at mealtime, will be the food in your stomach. I recommend that systemic enzyme supplements be taken at least one hour before or two hours after eating. I also suggest drinking at least eight ounces of water with the enzymes to facilitate their passage through the stomach.

Two to four tablets or capsules twice daily are adequate to control chronic inflammation and to allow the body to repair the microtrauma associated with physical exercise. Six tablets or capsules three times daily are often required to speed resolution of injuries or to bring improvement in conditions such as arthritis. As many as ten tablets or capsules four times daily have been used for management of severe injuries and major inflammatory conditions.

A change in color, consistency, and odor of stools occurs occasionally, but these effects are harmless. A few individuals have reported nausea or diarrhea, conditions that resolved by lowering the dosage or distributing it into numerous doses throughout the day.

It is recommended that individuals with a blood-clotting disturbance avoid systemic enzymes. People who are taking blood thinners such as Coumadin or platelet drugs such as aspirin should monitor their situation closely when introducing systemic enzyme supplements as the medication dosage may need to be lowered. Enzyme supplements should be discontinued 48 hours prior to major surgery, but they may be started immediately following the procedure and can significantly decrease post-operative pain and accelerate the healing process.

Mr. Itis can be controlled, and doing so can dramatically extend life while improving the quality of life in the process. Calming down Mr. Itis is one of the most significant steps that can be taken to improve the chances of living a long life free of degenerative conditions that make it difficult or impossible to pursue enjoyable activities. It is an issue that must be faced in reaching the goal of optimum wellness . . . dying young as late in life as possible.

Chapter 8

Support Your Internal Handyman

A wicked messenger falls into trouble, But a faithful ambassador brings health.
— Proverbs 13:17

———————————————— ❧ ————————————————

Free radical damage and inflammation cause damage to cell membranes, DNA, and other body tissues that, if unaddressed, can accelerate the aging process and lead to heart attacks, cancer, and degenerative diseases. Fortunately, the body is able to repair much of the damage before it becomes permanent. It does so by using molecules called methyl groups, which are the body's duct tape or super glue.

The body is based upon the chemical carbon. Methyl groups are among the simplest carbon molecules. As such, they are used in an infinite number of chemical reactions in the body. They are also key elements in the body's maintenance and repair processes. When the body runs low on methyl groups and their supporting cast, aging accelerates and degenerative diseases appear.

The Significance of Homocysteine

Fortunately it is possible to determine whether or not the body has adequate supplies of these critical nutrients. When the body runs low on methyl groups or the vitamins and minerals required for their use, a chemical called homocysteine accumulates. The level of homocysteine in the bloodstream can be measured, and that level is a direct reflection of the body's ability to maintain and repair itself.

Keith Mullen is one of the leading homocysteine researchers in the United States. His interest in homocysteine arose from personal experience.

Keith had his first heart attack when he was only forty-four years old. Although his total cholesterol of less than 200 and his cholesterol-to-HDL ratio of less than 4 indicated that he should be at low risk for heart disease, his cardiologist recommended that he reduce his cholesterol further. He was also advised to lose weight even though he was 5' 6" tall and weighed only 132 pounds.

His second heart attack occurred nine years later. His cholesterol was less than 200, his risk ratio less than 4, and his weight less than 135 pounds. Once again his cardiologist recommended that he lower his cholesterol and lose weight.

When he was advised to lower his cholesterol and lose weight following his third heart attack at age fifty-four, Keith concluded that something was missing in the doctor's recommendations. He began to look for other factors that might account for his proclivity to heart attacks.

Elevated levels of homocysteine, he discovered, dramatically increase one's risk of having a heart attack. He found his homocysteine level to be 58 mmol/L, making him over twelve times more likely than the average person to suffer a heart attack.

Keith began supplementing B vitamins, but he was only able to lower his homocysteine to 27 mmol/L, still far above the 6 or 7 that is generally regarded as safe. Addition of N-acetyl cysteine dropped his homocysteine into the safe range. He has not had a heart attack in the fifteen years since doing so.

Nearly everyone in the United States knows what cholesterol is and most can quote their cholesterol number. In contrast, relatively few people have heard of homocysteine and it is rare to find an individual who knows his or her homocysteine level.

Homocysteine is an amino acid. Amino acids are the building blocks from which proteins are made, and many amino acids are essential to health. Homocysteine, however, is toxic, damaging the walls of arteries and triggering the deposition of plaque. It is also known to induce DNA damage and accelerate cell death.

Detecting an increased risk of direct homocysteine toxicity may not be the most important reason for checking homocysteine levels, however. Researchers are beginning to realize that elevated levels of homocysteine often reflect the body's inability to perform ongoing maintenance and repair through a process called methylation.

The Methylation Process

Although most people have never heard the term, methylation is extremely important. Biochemically, it is the transfer of a methyl group, which is comprised of one carbon atom and three hydrogen atoms (CH3), from one molecule to another. Practically, it is the process the body uses to manufacture critical hormones like adrenaline and melatonin, to tell genes when to exert their influence, to detoxify foreign substances in the liver, to manufacture new cells, and to repair free radical damage.

Homocysteine forms when methionine, an amino acid obtained from various foods, is used as a source of methyl groups. Diet does not play a major role in the process, however. It has been demonstrated that dietary intakes of methionine up to five times that typically consumed do not cause homocysteine levels to rise. The primary reason levels rise is a loss of methylation capacity.

When the body's methylation reserve is adequate, homocysteine is converted to glutathione, an important antioxidant, or back to methionine. When the body's methylation reserve is inadequate or methylation does not proceed normally, homocysteine accumulates. Methylation deficiencies are associated with nearly every degenerative condition known. Rising homocysteine levels are found in heart disease, Alzheimer's disease, Parkinson's disease, multiple sclerosis, liver disease, depression, birth defects, cancer, premature aging, and other chronic illnesses.

It is difficult to find a condition that is not linked to inadequate methylation. An analysis of elderly hospitalized patients in France, published in 2003, showed that 100 percent had unsafe levels of homocysteine.[17] A startling 45 percent had levels above 15 mmol/L. A three-year study of elderly hospitalized patients in Italy, published in 2001, found that the mean homocysteine level was 16.8.[18] Patients with the highest levels tended to present with the most serious diseases and had the highest incidence of atherosclerosis and impaired mental function.

Homocysteine and Heart Attacks

Analysis of homocysteine levels in population subgroups is revealing. Individuals who are receiving dialysis treatments have some of the highest homocysteine levels of any group, often above 50. They also have one of the highest rates of heart attack.

An article published in the December 18, 2003 issue of the *New England Journal of Medicine* found the same to be true concerning a disease called Systemic Lupus Erythematous (SLE), often referred to simply as "lupus."[19] People who have SLE often die prematurely from a heart attack. The study found no increase in cholesterol or cholesterol risk ratios in lupus patients. What it did find was a significant increase in homocysteine levels.

In contrast, people with Down's syndrome have lower homocysteine levels than the general population, averaging between 2 and 3. This is due to the fact that a gene that regulates homocysteine metabolism is located on chromosome 21, an extra copy of which is carried by these individuals. While heart birth defects are common in Down's syndrome, heart attacks are not. I could find only one reported instance of an individual with Down's syndrome having a heart attack.

A study of the cholesterol patterns of people with Down's syndrome reveals something very interesting. The prevailing attitude is that high levels of cholesterol and LDL cholesterol (the so-called "bad" cholesterol) and low levels of HDL cholesterol (the so-called "good" cholesterol) cause heart attacks. Individuals with Down's syndrome have cholesterol and LDL levels that are no different than those in the general population and actually have LOWER than average levels of HDL cholesterol.[20] If the cholesterol and heart disease theory is correct, people with Down's syndrome should be having more heart attacks than the rest of the population, not less.

How rising homocysteine levels promote heart attacks is well-documented. Homocysteine is toxic to the lining of arteries. As homocysteine levels rise, injury to arterial walls increases. When injury occurs, the body sends a white blood cell called a macrophage to the site. Macrophage literally means "big eater." The job of the macrophage is to remove foreign substances from circulation, so that the risk of further injury is diminished. One of the substances viewed as "foreign" is oxidized LDL cholesterol.

LDL cholesterol, the so-called "bad" cholesterol, is harmless in its natural state. When it is attacked by a free radical and "oxidized," its appearance is changed. When a macrophage sees an oxidized LDL cholesterol particle floating by, it assumes it is a dangerous foreign substance. The "big eater" jumps into action, engulfing the oxidized LDL and pulling it into the wall of the artery. A macrophage containing oxidized LDL cholesterol is called a foam cell, and it is the first stage in the development of an atherosclerotic plaque.

The concept is quite simple: No injury to an artery wall, no plaque. No plaque, no heart attack. Lower homocysteine levels: less injury, less plaque. Higher homocysteine levels: more injury, more plaque.

It is therefore disappointing that the American Heart Association states, "The American Heart Association has not yet called hyperhomocysteinemia (high homocysteine level in the blood) a major risk factor for cardiovascular disease. We don't recommend widespread use of folic acid and B vitamin supplements to reduce the risk of heart disease and stroke."[21]

Homocysteine and Other Conditions

A clear and strong correlation of homocysteine levels to Alzheimer's Disease has also been discovered. Studies in the *International Journal of Geriatric Psychiatry*, April 1998,[22] and the Journal of Gerontology and Biological Sciences, March 1997,[23] confirmed that people with Alzheimer's disease have much higher homocysteine levels than others in their age group. A number of similar studies have confirmed the link.

Despite the mounting evidence that high levels of homocysteine are associated with Alzheimer's disease, I have been unable to find any Alzheimer's Disease support organization that encourages homocysteine testing and comprehensive nutritional supplementation to address the issue.

The American Heart Association and the Alzheimer's Disease Society are not alone in their resistance to homocysteine testing. Medicare excludes homocysteine screening as a benefit. The official Medicare position is that homocysteine testing is "not medically necessary." Skeptics take the position that any link between homocysteine and disease is unproven. They point to studies that appear to be inconclusive. These studies typically compare homocysteine levels in people having a particular disease with the levels in a control group of people without the disease, using a "normal" cutoff of up to 15 mmol/L. These studies err in failing to recognize an important fact: there is no "normal" level of homocysteine.

The *American Journal of Epidemiology* reported in 1996 that for each 3-point rise in homocysteine the risk of heart attack jumps 35 percent.[24] In 2008, the Mayo Clinic published a review of twenty-six studies of homocysteine levels, heart disease risk factors, and coronary artery disease (heart attacks).[25] The researchers found a 20 – 50 percent increase in heart attack risk for every 5-point increase in the homocysteine blood level. This was independent of other commonly accepted risk factors. Other studies looking at the incidence of disease at progressively rising homocysteine levels have shown similar results.

Studies comparing people who have had a heart attack or have developed Alzheimer's disease with the population at large have reported inconclusive results. This is not surprising when one considers that the average homocysteine level of people living in the United States is 10 mmol/L. Since a rise in homocysteine from 6.5 mmol/L to 10 mmol/L increases the risk of heart attack by 35 percent, many researchers are actually comparing people who have had a heart attack with people who are likely to have a heart attack. No wonder their results are "inconclusive." One must compare the disease incidence in individuals with high levels of homocysteine with that in those with low levels to draw a logical conclusion.

Over fifteen hundred articles linking elevated homocysteine levels with diseases of the circulatory system have been published in major medical journals. Not only do high homocysteine levels reflect an increased risk for heart attacks, but they are also associated with the risk of stroke, peripheral vascular disease, dissecting aortic aneurysm, congestive heart failure, cardiomyopathy (an enlarged heart), venous thrombosis (blood clots), and retinal vein occlusion (a stroke affecting vision).

Elevated homocysteine levels are found in most diseases of the nervous system, including Alzheimer's Disease, vascular dementia, Parkinson's Disease, multiple sclerosis, and epilepsy. When they are present in hepatitis C, a greater incidence of scarring is found. Cirrhosis of the liver, kidney failure, diabetic complications, osteoporosis, and auto-immune diseases are also characterized by high levels of homocysteine.

Rising homocysteine levels are found in nearly all complications of pregnancy, including miscarriage, premature delivery, toxemia, and stillbirth. High levels predispose to birth defects, including neural tube defects (a failure of the spine to close), heart defects, and Down's syndrome. (People with Down's syndrome have very low homocysteine levels, but a high homocysteine level in a woman prior to pregnancy increases the risk of her baby having Down's syndrome.)

Many cancers have been shown to be associated with elevated homocysteine. Some of these are cancers of the breast, cervix, colon, head and neck, and stomach.

Supporting Methylation

If it were not possible to support methylation and control homocysteine levels, the reluctance of physicians and organizations to accept the link between homocysteine and degenerative diseases might be understandable. The truth, however, is that elevated homocysteine levels can be reduced easily, safely, and inexpensively.

Several lifestyle factors can be addressed. Consuming more than two alcoholic beverages daily, smoking cigarettes, and drinking over nine cups of coffee daily have been shown to trigger a rise in homocysteine. Following a vegan diet and performing physical activity regularly will tend to lower one's homocysteine level. In most cases, however, nutritional supplementation will be needed to effectively bring homocysteine into a safe range of 7.2 mmol/L or less. This is because the processes that determine homocysteine utilization or elimination are dependent upon nutrients that are often deficient in the American diet.

Three mechanisms are involved in maintaining safe homocysteine levels. The first is called remethylation, which is the process of combining a methyl group with homocysteine to form the amino acids methionine or S-adenostyl methionine (SAM-e). This requires folic acid, B12, zinc, and a methyl donor such as dimethylglycine or trimethylglycine.

The second is called trans-sulfuration, which involves changing the location of a sulfur atom. This converts homocysteine to a useful amino acid, cysteine, or to glutathione, an important antioxidant. Trans-sulfuration requires vitamin B6 and magnesium.

The third means of handling homocysteine is to excrete it from the body through the kidneys. This process is greatly enhanced by the presence of a substance called N-acetylcysteine.

The Role of Nutritional Supplementation

The benefit of supplementation with the nutrients that support those mechanisms has been demonstrated conclusively. B6 (pyridoxine) deficiency was reported to increase the risk of atherosclerosis (hardening of the arteries) in monkeys in 1949.[26] The relationship of B6 deficiency to human atherosclerosis was confirmed in 1951.[27] Homocysteine damage to arteries in individuals with low B6 levels was noted in 1969.[28]

Two observational reports confirm the benefit of B6 supplementation in reducing heart attack risk. In 1950, Dr. Moses Suzman, a neurologist in Johannesburg, South Africa, began recommending that his patients take 200 mg. of B6 daily. He made this recommendation to thousands of people over the course of his career. Dr. Suzman subsequently reported that over a period of 44 years he did not learn of a single heart attack, cardiac arrest, or stroke in those patients—even those with high blood pressure.[29] It is likely that some heart attacks or strokes occurred, but the fact that Dr. Suzman was unaware of any suggests that the incidence of those events was lower than would be expected.

In 1962, Dr. John Ellis, a family physician in Mount Pleasant, Texas, began treating carpal tunnel syndrome with 50 – 200 mg. of vitamin B6 daily. He published his experience with those patients in 1995. When Dr. Ellis analyzed his practice he found that those patients taking vitamin B6 had one-fourth the number of heart attacks of his other patients. He also noted that when elderly patients died at home (usually of a presumed heart attack), they did so eight years later than those who had not been treated with B6.[30]

An inverse relationship between levels of vitamin B12 and homocysteine was reported in 1988.[31] Further, an increased risk of heart attack for individuals with low B12 levels was documented in 1995.[32]

High homocysteine levels were found to be associated with low folic acid levels in 1987.[33] The risk of birth defects due to low folic acid levels was postulated in 1994[34] and the benefit of folic acid supplementation in preventing those birth defects was reported in 1996.[35] As a result, several foods are now fortified with folic acid.

Additionally, the role of zinc in the methylation process was shown in animal studies published in 1985.[36] The fact that human betaine-homocysteine transferase, an important enzyme in the methylation process, is dependent upon the presences of zinc was recognized and reported in 1998.[37]

A connection between low magnesium levels and heart attack risk was reported in 1977;[38] a similar relationship with peripheral vascular disease was reported in 1990.[39]

Individuals receiving dialysis for management of kidney failure have extremely high homocysteine levels. If they do not die from their kidney disease, they are very likely to die of a heart attack. The benefit of trimethylglycine in reducing homocysteine in dialysis patients was reported in 2002.[40] Next, the fact that the benefit extended to people who do not have kidney failure was noted in 2005.[41]

The effectiveness of N-acetylcysteine (NAC) supplementation in lowering homocysteine levels was first reported in 1996[42], and long-term effectiveness was confirmed in 2003.[43] This is because the NAC-homocysteine complex is cleared by the kidneys much more effectively than is homocysteine alone.

The importance of taking a comprehensive approach to lowering homocysteine levels was pointed out in a 2008 editorial that accompanied a Mayo Clinic article on homocysteine and heart attack risk.[44] Noting that B vitamins alone are ineffective in reducing the risk of heart attack in those with elevated homocysteine levels, the commentator called for yet-to-be-developed pharmacologic therapies and combinations of methionine restriction, exercise, and use of betaine-homocysteine methyltransferase and N-acetylcysteine in addressing the problem of high homocysteine blood levels. In effect, the editorial recommended the use of the nutrient combination found in *HCY Formula*, a methylation support product I had developed several years earlier.

Those who suggest that people should wait to lower homocysteine until the results of long-term studies conclusively prove the consequences of ineffective methylation to everyone's satisfaction are in a state of deep denial. The connection between Vitamin B-6 and heart disease was reported as early as 1948 and the connection between B-12 deficiencies and dementia was reported in 1969. The homocysteine connection was recognized as early as 1980.

If you do not know your homocysteine level, I encourage you to have it checked immediately, and, if it is over 7, take steps to bring it into a safer range. Because the body's methylation capacity tends to diminish with age and can fall off quickly, everyone over the age of 70 should check his or her homocysteine level annually.

The mechanisms that trigger and direct the aging process are complex, but a great deal has been learned in the past two decades. It has become clear that methylation is the primary mechanism the body uses to repair free radical damage and that homocysteine levels are a reliable indicator of the body's ability or inability to perform maintenance and repair tasks. By providing nutrients that support the repair of the damage to cell membranes, DNA, and other body components as it occurs, each of us can expect to age gracefully and die biologically young at an advanced chronological age.

Chapter 9
Put the Pedal to the Metal

Those who wait on the Lord shall renew their strength;
They shall mount up with wings like eagles,
They shall run and not be weary.
They shall walk and not faint.
– Isaiah 40:31

Catching a "Second Wind"

Runners are familiar with a phenomenon called "catching a second wind." It describes the experience of having reached a point in the run where one is gasping for breath and has to slow down. Many find that after a few seconds they feel recovered and are able to once again pick up the pace.

While exercise physiologists do not agree on what accounts for the phenomenon, there is no doubt about its existence. The body, it seems, has the ability to increase energy production when demand requires that it do so. A young, physically fit person is likely to reach the point of gasping for air only with intense exertion. Older individuals or those with conditions that limit their ability to supply oxygen to their cells often experience shortness of breath or labored breathing at much lower levels of activity. No matter at what level it appears, all who experience air hunger long to catch a "second wind"—to be able to perform at a higher level for a longer period of time.

Shortness of breath occurs when the body is not receiving the amount of oxygen required to meet its energy needs. The obvious answer to providing a second wind is to increase the amount of oxygen available. This is generally accomplished by breathing air containing a higher percentage of oxygen. It is not uncommon to see a football player breathing from an oxygen tank along the sidelines following a long run, nor is it unusual to see a person with emphysema or heart failure using an oxygen tank as he or she attempts to ease the shortness of breath experienced with routine daily activities.

An alternative to oxygen administration as a means to provide a second wind exists. Increasing the efficiency of oxygen utilization by the body can be as effective as, and in some cases more effective than, providing additional oxygen.

Energy Production in the Body

Every cell of the body comes equipped with power plants called mitochondria. Cells with high energy demand, such as heart muscle cells, may contain thousands of mitochondria. Cells with low energy needs may contain a few dozen. Mitochondrial energy production is absolutely essential for producing physical strength and stamina and for sustaining life. Even a slight drop in energy output can lead to weakness, fatigue, and difficulty concentrating.

The body is equipped with three energy producing methods. Under most circumstances, energy is produced by what is called aerobic (oxygen dependent) metabolism. The level of activity that can be performed aerobically is determined by several factors. These include the volume of air moving in and out of the lungs, the efficiency of oxygen exchange between the alveoli (lung air sacs) and the hemoglobin molecule in red blood cells, the effectiveness of the heart in circulating blood throughout the body, and the ability of mitochondria, the energy-producing factories of cells, to function efficiently.

Breathing correctly by making full use of the diaphragm to move air is the first step in increasing one's capacity to perform physical activities. In circumstances where the amount of available oxygen is low, such as living at a high altitude, the body will respond by manufacturing a greater number of red blood cells to improve the exchange rate. Regular physical activity can significantly improve the heart's ability to pump blood throughout the body. In addition, the needs of the mitochondria can be supported nutritionally.

When the amount of oxygen supplied to mitochondria is insufficient to meet the body's energy needs, the mitochondria can implement the second method of energy production, which is anaerobic (non-oxygen dependent) metabolism. Increasing the volume of air moved, improving oxygen uptake by the red blood cells, and enhancing circulation will not boost anaerobic metabolism significantly. Supporting mitochondrial function can, however, increase anaerobic capacity.

The third method of producing energy is called the phosphagen system. This method of energy production is of very limited capacity and can only be maintained for approximately 8 to 10 seconds. It is beneficial to allow sudden exertion, but it cannot be relied upon to supply energy for sustained activity. Little, if anything, can be done to increase the efficiency of the phosphagen system.

The energy source common to all three methods is a substance called adenosine triphosphate (ATP). ATP is made up of one adenosine molecule to which three phosphate ions are attached. ATP contains large amounts of potential energy. This energy is released when phosphate ions are separated from ATP to produce either ADP (an adenosine with two phosphate ions attached) or AMP (an adenosine molecule with one phosphate attached).

When the body is relying upon the phosphagen system for energy production, it is burning the ATP that is immediately available in its cells and ATP that can be created quickly from a substance called creatine phosphate. (Creatine phosphate is a naturally occurring substance and should not be confused with the creatine supplements advocated by some body builders.) Since cells can store limited amounts of ATP and creatine phosphate, the ability to produce energy in this manner is extremely limited.

The Lactic Acid Threshold

Cells contain larger quantities of glycogen, a source of glucose that can be used to produce ATP without the use of oxygen. Glycogen stores are generally adequate to produce enough ATP to supply energy needs for approximately one and a half minutes. A byproduct of the conversion of glycogen to ATP in this manner is a substance called lactic acid.

Lactic acid is used to produce more ATP and fuel muscular activity. As long as adequate amounts of oxygen are available, it is burned completely for energy or converted to glycogen for energy storage. When oxygen demands cannot be met, however, lactic acid accumulates. The build-up of lactic acid in muscles causes them to become stiff and sore, forcing a decrease in the intensity of the activity. The point at which lactic acid begins to accumulate is referred to as the lactic acid threshold.

As mitochondrial energy production becomes more efficient, the lactic acid threshold will rise. This can be increased by regularly participating in physical activities that push the body's limits. This is why distance runners can improve their performance by incorporating short sprints into their training regimen. Supporting mitochondrial nutritional needs can augment the benefits of physical training.

Mitochondrial Supports

One of the first mitochondrial supports to be introduced was ubiquinone, more commonly known as coenzyme Q10. Discovered in 1957, coenzyme Q10 is critical to the production of ATP. It acts as a transporter of electrons in the critical reactions that allow mitochondria to produce energy.

Coenzyme Q10 is manufactured by the body, but production begins to decline around the age of thirty and levels continue to fall as people age. Deficiencies of coenzyme Q10 are associated with a number of conditions, including congestive heart failure, muscular dystrophy, gingivitis, and cancer. Supplementation of coenzyme Q10 is capable of producing dramatic results.

The severity of heart disease is commonly defined by determining an individual's capacity to perform activity. Four functional classes exist. People with Class I disease are able to perform ordinary activities without difficulty. Those with Class II disease are comfortable at rest or with mild exertion, but cannot do many common activities, such as climbing stairs or walking across a parking lot, without experiencing shortness of breath or excessive fatigue. Class III disease is characterized by marked limitation of activity. Comfort is achieved only by remaining at rest. Individuals with Class IV disease are prone to symptoms such as shortness of breath even at rest and are unable to perform any physical activity.

In a University of Texas study involving 424 patients, 58 percent improved by one functional class, 28 percent by two classes, and 1 – 2 percent by three activity classes when given coenzyme Q10! Nearly 90 percent of them experienced a significant improvement in their quality of life. Not only were they able to significantly increase their physical activity, 43 percent were able to stop taking between one and three prescription drugs![45]

Consider what those results mean to individuals with heart disease. A one class improvement, achieved by over half of those taking coenzyme Q10, will allow a Class IV individual to go from being uncomfortable at rest to being completely free of symptoms at rest. A person with a Class II disability is able to resume normal activity. Imagine the experience of the individuals who move up three functional classes. Those people go from being uncomfortable at rest to being able to perform normal activities with ease!

L-carnitine is another nutrient that is helpful in improving energy production. L-carnitine is responsible for carrying fats, such as triglycerides, into the mitochondria where they can be converted to energy. This is important in all muscles, but it is especially important in the heart, since the heart relies more heavily upon fatty acids as its energy source than do other tissues. L-carnitine has been shown to improve recovery after intense exercise and to improve stamina and exercise capacity in people with ischemic heart disease.[46] As beneficial as coenzyme Q10 or L-carnitine have proven to be for individuals with compromised mitochondrial function when given separately, the combination of the two often brings about even greater improvement.

Two other nutrients that have shown the ability to work together to support mitochondrial function are alpha ketoglutaric acid and L-malic acid. When anaerobic (low oxygen) conditions exist, these substances enhance the production of a chemical called succinate. When oxygen becomes available, the mitochondria are able to use succinate to bypass a rate-limiting step and rapidly increase the aerobic production of ATP. This translates into a more rapid recovery when oxygen levels are restored.

Increased succinate levels are believed to enhance athletic performance. Improved succinate availability has also been shown to reverse cases of respiratory failure and a condition known as MELAS (mitochondrial encephalopathy, lactic acidosis, and stroke-like episodes).[47] Supplementation of alpha ketoglutaric acid and malic acid appears to be one of the most effective ways to increase mitochondrial succinate levels.[48]

Alpha lipoic acid is receiving increasing attention as a mitochondrial support nutrient. Best known for its effectiveness as an antioxidant, alpha lipoic acid plays a significant role in mitochondrial production of ATP. Animal studies have demonstrated that it can reverse age-related mitochondrial decline. Activity levels in older animals, which were initially one-third that of younger counterparts, were significantly increased by alpha lipoic acid supplementation.[49] In a separate study, the mitochondrial activity of liver cells, which declined in non-supplemented animals, remained steady in those receiving alpha lipoic acid.[50]

Another substance, inosine, is believed to enhance mitochondrial energy production and improve the delivery of oxygen to body tissues. Claims associated with inosine supplementation have included increased energy levels, improved endurance, enhanced ATP production, increased oxygen delivery to tissues, reduced lactic acid accumulation in muscles, and improved muscle development.

Inosine is a building block of adenosine, the core molecule of ATP. It facilitates the use of carbohydrate by the heart muscle, making heart muscle less vulnerable to low oxygen states. Inosine also increases levels of 2,3-DPG, a compound found in red blood cells.[51] 2,3-DPG enhances the release of oxygen from the red cells to the body tissues. In addition, it improves the removal of excess lactic acid from muscle cells.

While studies have not demonstrated an improvement in aerobic performance, inosine has been extensively used by world-class power lifters and other strength athletes in Russia and the other former Eastern Bloc countries to increase their bodies' oxygen-carrying capacity and improve muscle contraction. Inosine's primary benefits relate to its ability to increase the body's ability to handle strenuous exercise, intense training programs, and competitive events. By improving muscular energy production and the ability of red blood cells to transport oxygen, recovery times are significantly shortened. Inosine has anti-inflammatory effects, which may account for the finding that less muscle soreness and stiffness is experienced after intense muscular activity when it is a part of the training regimen.

Inosine is also being shown to be protective against nerve damage. It has been patented as a treatment for stroke, as inosine supplementation has been shown to facilitate the rewiring of the brain after injury.[52] Studies of its effectiveness in slowing the progression of multiple sclerosis are promising.[53]

Mitochondrial Decline and Disease

Clearly, mitochondrial efficiency is critical to muscular performance and recovery from intense activity. Loss of mitochondrial function accounts for much of the loss of energy and vitality typically associated with aging. In addition, mitochondrial dysfunction is believed to play a role in the development of many diseases. Some include Parkinson's disease, Alzheimer's disease, multiple sclerosis, amylotrophic lateral sclerosis (Lou Gehrig's disease), Huntington's disease, muscular dystrophy, drug-induced myopathy, myasthenia gravis, autism, attention deficit disorder, depression, bipolar disorder, cancer, metabolic syndrome, type 2 diabetes, atherosclerosis, ischemic heart disease, congestive heart failure, cardiomyopathy, non-alcoholic fatty liver disease, asthma, COPD (emphysema), migraine, fibromyalgia, and chronic fatigue syndromes.

The leading cause of mitochondrial dysfunction is believed to be oxidative damage. Because of its ability to maintain levels of glutathione, an important mitochondrial antioxidant, N-acetyl cysteine (NAC) helps maintain mitochondrial integrity. Animals supplemented with NAC maintained significantly higher mitochondrial function over time than non-supplemented controls. The NAC also protected cells from premature death.[54] Ginkgo biloba is believed to prevent age-associated memory loss by this same mechanism.

Omega-3 fish oils have also been shown to be helpful in preventing age-related decline in mitochondrial function. This is now believed to be the major reason that omega-3 supplements protect heart function during aging and make the heart muscle less susceptible to damage from ischemia (lack of oxygen).

Mitochondrial dysfunction is recognized as a significant factor in the aging process and the development of degenerative diseases. Supporting your body's energy factories can dramatically expand your ability to perform physical activities in the present while helping you age gracefully in the future.

Chapter 10
What You Can't See Can Kill You!

*The opinion of 10,000 men is of no value if none of them
know anything about the subject.*
– Marcus Aurelius

Rising Disease Incidence

We live in a dangerous world. We are threatened by natural disasters such as earthquakes, tornados, hurricanes, and blizzards. We can just as easily fall victim to microbes too small to be seen by the naked eye such as viruses, bacteria, fungi, and protozoa. We may suffer physical injury as a result of our own actions or those of others. One can die as swiftly by falling off one's own roof as by being hit by a drunk driver or blown to bits by a terrorist.

There are also unseen and generally unrecognized hazards. While we pride ourselves on ridding the environment of second-hand smoke and turning our societal attention to the elimination of trans-fats in prepared foods, we are willfully ignoring more real and present dangers. It is quite likely that we are in the process of demonstrating that suicide is just as deadly if committed as a civilization as it is when one person takes his or her own life.

There has been a dramatic change in disease incidence over the past half-century. It is also clear that the rate of change is accelerating. In 1955, the lifetime risk of cancer was one in twelve. One out of every twelve people in the United States could expect to develop cancer at some point in his or her life. This would almost always be late in onset—in one's sixties, seventies, or eighties. By 2000, I began telling audiences that the lifetime cancer risk stood at one in four and was expected to reach one in three by the end of the decade.

I was wrong. Very wrong! According to the SEER Cancer Statistics Review released by the National Cancer Institute in April 2006, the lifetime risk of developing cancer was closer to one in two (47 percent for men and 42 percent for women). This estimate was based upon data collected from 2001 to 2003 (the most recent years for which statistics were available). This means that while we *thought* the risk of developing cancer at the turn of the twenty-first century was one in four it was *actually* one in two!

The good news is that the risk of developing cancer has remained stable over the past several years. The statistics for 2007, released in 2010 showed a lifetime risk of 46 percent in men and 42 percent in women[55]. We do not know, however, what the future holds. In a 2000 interview with reporter Linda Howe, Dr. Robert Becker, a pioneer in electromagnetic medicine who has been following the increasing incidence of cancer and other diseases, suggested that it is not unreasonable to expect the lifetime risk of cancer to reach 100 percent or even 200 percent—two cancers per person.

Another disease process that is increasing in frequency is Alzheimer's disease. First identified one hundred years ago and relatively rare in the mid-twentieth century, it has risen to the seventh leading cause of death in the United States. In November 2006 the *Los Angeles Times* reported that the death rate from Alzheimer's disease in Los Angeles County had risen an astounding 220 percent in the decade between 1994 and 2003.[56] The report was based upon statistics released by the Los Angeles Health Department.

Attention Deficit Disorder did not exist in 1950. It was rare in the 1970s. Today it is present in epidemic proportions. Ten percent of the United States' population is said to be affected.[57,58] One out of every three boys in some classrooms is classified as having ADD or ADHD, and girls are being diagnosed with increasing frequency.

Fibromyalgia syndrome, rarely described before 1975, was not officially declared a syndrome and accepted as a medical diagnosis until 1993. In its Copenhagen Declaration, the World Health Organization stated, "Fibromyalgia is part of a wider syndrome encompassing headaches, irritable bladder, dysmenorrhea, cold sensitivity, Reynaud's phenomenon, restless legs, atypical patterns of numbness and tingling, exercise intolerance, and complaints of weakness."[59] Depression was also mentioned as a common finding in individuals with the syndrome.

It is believed that up to 5 percent of the population of the United States is currently affected by fibromyalgia and some believe that one out of three people will experience its symptoms at some point during their lives.[60]

The prevalence of sleep disorders is currently felt to be one in six—approximately forty million people in the United States having sleep difficulty at any given time.[61] Restless legs syndrome, recognized but rare thirty years ago, is now believed to be present in approximately 8 – 12 percent of the U.S. populace, an increase of 5 – 9 percent over the past decade.[62]

It is possible to summarize the change in disease prevalence by stating that cancer and rheumatic, psychiatric, and neurological disorders have been occurring with increasing frequency since 1955 and that they have been rising exponentially since 1975. Attempts to explain this unprecedented rise in illness as due to "improved diagnosis and reporting," "poor eating habits," an "aging population," or "mass hysteria" cannot be taken seriously. Something is systematically destroying the integrity of the human body.

The Human Body and the Electromagnetic Spectrum

We live in an electromagnetic universe. The light we see is only a small portion of what is called the electromagnetic spectrum. You and I emit infrared energy that is slightly outside of the visible spectrum. Electromagnetic radiation consists of vibrations or waves. It is classified by wavelength (the distance from the peak of one wave to the peak of the next), frequency (speed), and energy level. On one end of the spectrum are gamma rays, which have short wavelengths, high frequency and high energy. At the other end are AM radio waves that have long wavelengths, low frequencies, and low energy (See Figure 1).

Radiation on the short wavelength, high-frequency side of the spectrum is referred to as ionizing radiation. Radiation of long wavelength and low frequency is called non-ionizing radiation. The most significant forms of non-ionizing radiation are radio frequencies and microwaves (RF/MW).

That ionizing radiation can damage living tissues and trigger disease is universally accepted by the medical community. On the other hand, the suggestion that non-ionizing radiation, such as FM radio and television broadcasts, cellular telephone signals, and computer WiFi networks, can cause harm is almost universally rejected. Nevertheless, I am convinced, beyond a shadow of doubt, that the unprecedented rise in cancer and diseases of the neuromuscular system

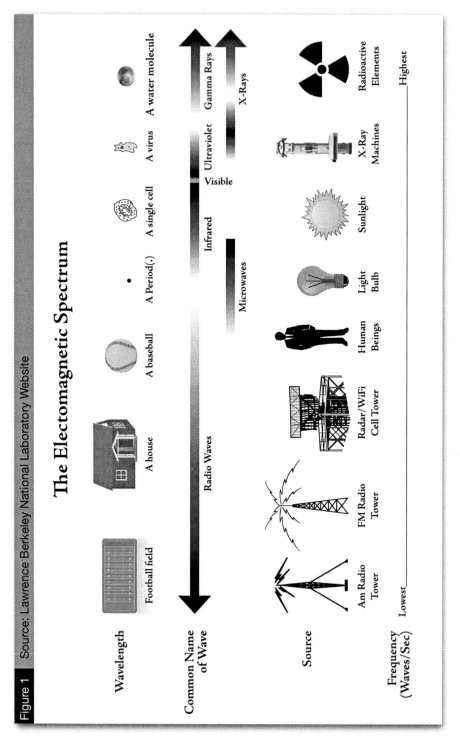

is due largely, if not exclusively, to the increased presence of RF/MW radiation in the environment.

I am aware that published studies in major journals overwhelmingly support the opinion that RF/MW is safe and has no effect upon human health. That does not surprise me. Researchers who report adverse effects from RF/MW lose their funding. Dr. Jerry Phillips, for example, received a research grant from Motorola Corporation. When he found evidence of damage caused by RF/MW radiation and reported his findings to Motorola, he was told that his work was not ready for publication. He was offered additional funding to continue his experiment (to "get it right!"). Phillips refused to cover up his data and did publish it, but his funding was cut off and he has not been able to do any additional RF/MW studies. Inexplicably, when Dr. Phillips's article appeared in print it concluded with the statement that while changes were observed, they were "probably of no physiological significance."[63]

The source of funding for RF/MW research is of grave concern given the marked difference in results of industry- or military-sponsored studies and those of independent researchers. While the number of published studies showing no DNA damage from RF/MW radiation is approximately equal to the number of studies that report DNA damage, the funding bias is immediately apparent. Eighty-five studies looking for DNA damage from exposure to RF/MW were conducted from 1990-2006. Forty-five reported negative effects and forty-two reported no adverse effects. Of the forty-five that found an association between RF/MW exposure and DNA damage, forty-two were privately funded and three were commissioned by industry. Thirty-seven of the forty-two studies that showed no ill effect were funded by industry. One of the remaining five studies showing no effect was conducted by an individual with industry ties who would not disclose his funding source.[64]

Similarly, a University of Washington analysis found that biological effects of RF/MW are reported in 81 percent of non-industry-funded studies, but in only 19 percent of those funded by industry—which, outside of the military, is the only source of funding today. When confronted with these statistics, Dr. Mays Swicord, director of electromagnetic research at Motorola, responded that industry funds quality work while independent research is "sloppy."[65]

When the work of researchers critical to RF/MW is cited, the authors are often referred to not as scientists, but as "scientists," the brackets giving the same implication for Ph.D.s as the word quack does for physicians. They are no longer real scientists; they are "scientists" who do not deserve the title, and their work is "controversial." Professor Henry Lai of the University of Washington, who was the first to demonstrate RF/MW-induced DNA damage, was subsequently threatened with litigation by an industry group, which also sought his firing by the university.[66]

Closely related to the loss of funding issue is the ability of RF/MW safety advocates to state that studies demonstrating an adverse effect have not been replicated. No funding, no research, no replication. Yet this charge is used regularly to discredit the original findings.

Industries that rely heavily upon radio wave or microwave technology liberally support individuals and institutions that publish studies that support the contention that the technologies are safe. It is not particularly difficult to design studies to achieve a predetermined or desired result. This may be happening in the area of RF/MW, as I have observed that whenever a study has been published that demonstrates an adverse effect of RF/MW, others soon follow to rebut the findings. This was almost certainly true in the case of the "Dead Mice Walking" study, which I will detail later.

There are many reasons why studies would fail to demonstrate that a problem exists. The most glaring miscalculation is the assumption that there are "safe" and "unsafe" levels of radiation. The overwhelming majority of studies compare the prevalence of disease in subjects who live close to a broadcast or cellular telephone tower to those living some distance away from the tower. Likewise, they may compare cell phone users to non-users. If, as independent research has shown, there is no "safe" level of RF/MW, the results of such studies are meaningless, as they are simply comparing one group of people who are being radiated with another group of people who are being radiated. Failing to find a difference in disease incidence does not prove that radiation is "safe" unless one assumes (and there is no basis upon which to do so) that only intense radiation has the capability of producing adverse effects.

One of the recurring arguments against funding research into the health effects of RF/MW is that "levels of microwave radiation used for cellular telephone or WiFi networks are well below the levels that are known to be safe." The industry is able to discount any health challenge perceived to be related to

RF/MW because "the level of radiation is one hundred times below the level that has been shown to be safe."

"Safe" levels of RF/MW radiation were set by determining, for example, how much RF/MW radiation is required to heat water in a balloon. The fact that the human body relies upon low-level electrical and magnetic gradients to maintain integrity and to carry on intercellular communication was never considered when "safe" levels were being established.

The assumption used in most RF/MW studies—that only the generation of heat will cause damage—is indefensible. The heat theory of safety was shown to be false by a Walter Reed Army Research program, which found that "microwave energy of the militarily significant range of 1 to 15 GHz enters into all organ systems of the body and therefore constitutes a danger to all organ systems."[67] (Cellular telephones operate in the 2.4 to 5.8 GHz range.)

The greatest difficulty, however, is investigative bias. Mark Twain cleverly quipped, "There are three types of lies: lies, damn lies, and statistics." His observation was profound—investigators can flip the conclusion of a study 180 degrees depending upon which form of statistical analysis they choose to apply. Later in this chapter I will contrast two studies that looked at exactly the same data. One, which gained publication in a United States journal, found a cluster of cancer cases to be completely random. The other, published in an obscure journal, used more sophisticated methods of analysis and found the relationship of the cancer cases to RF radiation to be so strong that the computer program could not calculate the odds of it occurring by chance.

Closely related to investigator bias is editorial bias, commonly referred to as "peer review." Journal editors review submitted papers, purportedly to weed out those that do not follow high research standards. In reality, journal editors arbitrarily select articles that support the position the journal wishes to promote.

A prime example of editorial bias is the journal *Radiation Research*. The July 2006 issue of *Microwave News* carried the results of an investigation into *Radiation Research*'s editorial record.[68] Between 1991 and 2007, *Radiation Research* published only one paper that showed an adverse effect of RF/MW. In contrast, the journal carried twenty-one articles that claimed that RF/MW radiation does not cause any adverse effects. (The author of the only adverse study published lost her funding and was forced to move to a different line of research.)

While the editors of *Radiation Research* contend that they are publishing based upon quality rather than study conclusions, the evidence suggests otherwise. One of the studies *Radiation Research* chose to publish has come to be known as "Dead Mice Walking."[69] Supported by Motorola, the study was published soon after an independent study had shown an increased cancer rate in mice exposed to RF/MW radiation. The study is widely used today to support the contention that RF/MW radiation is harmless, but mice that were shown to have died at one point in the study were still being counted and weighed in another.

The last two decades have seen a dramatic increase in RF/MW radiation. We have seen the introduction of high-speed cellular communication networks, WiFi hot spots, Bluetooth connectivity, satellite radio broadcasting, GPS guidance systems, Doppler radar, portable phones, radiofrequency identification (RFID) systems for inventory control, and WiMax. The total effect that RF/MW expansion will have on human health is as yet unknown, but the outlook is ominous.

Can a Honey Bee Be a Canary?

Coal mining is a dangerous occupation. Underground mining hazards include suffocation from inadequate ventilation, gas poisoning, roof collapse, and explosions. Before the advent of electronic warning systems, miners would take a canary with them as they descended into the mine. This is because canaries are particularly sensitive to the presence of poisonous gasses such as methane and carbon monoxide. As long as the canary was singing, the miners knew that the air was safe to breathe. If the canary stopped singing, however, the miners knew that they must exit the mine immediately.

The rapid expanse of cellular communication networks was aided in the United States by the passage of the Telecommunications Act of 1996. Section 704 a, subsection D states, *"State or Local Governments May Not Regulate Wireless Facilities on the Basis of Environmental Effects of Radio Frequency Emissions if the Applicant Demonstrates Compliance with FCC Regulations."*

The rule was put in place to eliminate debate concerning health issues when a permit for placement of a cell phone tower was requested at the local level. Congress obviously believed that microwave radiation exposure was harmless and that individuals expressing concern about the adverse effects of microwave radiation on the human body were "kooks" standing in the way of progress. (Bear in mind that the same government that prohibits discussion of the effects of cell phones on the human body requires that cell phones and other electronic devices be turned off during the take-off and landing of commercial aircraft so that their frequencies do not interfere with the proper functioning of instruments in the cockpit.)

Over the past three and a half years there has been a dramatic decline in the honey bee population in the United States and around the world. This is a serious phenomenon, since at least 30 percent of food crops require cross-pollination facilitated by honey bees to produce fruit.

Honey bee losses began being reported in October 2006. It was initially hoped that this was an isolated phenomenon due to weather or an unknown, but self-limiting, disease process. As losses continued to mount, however, a new term was coined—colony collapse disorder (CCD).

Colony collapse disorder is a phenomenon that is new to bee-keeping. The disorder is characterized by empty hives, not hives filled with dead bees. This is significant because if the bees were dying from a parasitic or viral infection one would expect many of them to die in the hive. In CCD the worker bees appear to have left the hive in search of honey and have failed to return.

Historically, occasional bees would fail to return to the hive, but in CCD all of the worker bees fail to return, resulting in the death of the unsupported queen and immature bees that were left behind.

Many theories have been advanced to explain the appearance of CCD. Some of these include infection of the bees by parasites, mites or other pathogens, poor nutrition, global warming (climate change), and high stress levels among adult bees. The last theory, while creative, is patently ridiculous. Those proposing the "high stress" theory argue that the expansion of agriculture has created larger and more numerous fields that have forced the bees to overwork. While we humans may be guilty of placing unreasonable demands upon ourselves, I find it hard to believe that honey bees are surveying the size and number of fields and determining that they have to work overtime to complete the pollination task at hand.

There is a mechanism that explains the character and timing of colony collapse disorder. It is the rise of radiofrequency/microwave radiation levels in recent years. Honey bees rely upon information they receive from the earth's electromagnetic field to orient themselves and locate their hive once they have finished their task of collecting nectar for honey production. The energy levels produced by cellular networks are 10^{10} (10 followed by 10 zeros) times stronger than that of the earth's electromagnetic field. When a hive is located in operational proximity to a cell phone tower (meaning that cellular phone reception is present at the site) the microwave frequencies generated by the tower overpower the earth's electromagnetic field. This disables the bees' GPS system and leaves them wandering aimlessly in search of their home base.

This mechanism has been tested and found to be true.

One of the first studies looking at the effect of non-ionizing radiation on honey bees was conducted by the University of Koblenz in Landau, Germany. In 2006 they reported their findings that placing the base unit for a portable phone (the type commonly used in homes rather than a cell phone) in the hive prevented worker bees from returning to the hive.[70]

The Koblenz study was met with skepticism. The headline of an April 2007 article at *Der Spiegel Online* reads "Debunking a New Myth—Mobile Phones and Honey Bees."[71] Nothing in the body of the article disproved the theory; in fact, sources were quoted as saying the association was worthy of consideration and required more study.

More study has been done. One study was done by Sainuddeen Pattazhy, a researcher and dean in the department of zoology at SN College, Punalur, Kerala, India.[72] When Pattazhy and his colleagues placed mobile phones in proximity to beehives, the hives collapsed completely within five to ten days due to the failure of worker bees to return. Pattazhy explained the phenomenon in part by the phones' interference with the bees' navigation system, but he also noted that radiation exposure damages the bees' nervous system, resulting in a loss of the ability to fly.

Could the collapse of honey bee colonies be the equivalent of the canary in a coal mine that has stopped singing? I believe this question should be taken seriously. After all, Albert Einstein once observed, "If the bee disappeared off the surface of the globe then man would only have four years of life left. No more bees, no more pollination, no more plants, no more animals, no more man."

Not only may honey bees be in danger of extinction, canaries may well stop singing due to exposure to frequencies in the 900–1800 MHz range emitted by cellular towers. Professor Pattazhy has found that radiation from phone towers threatens the existence of sparrows and other small birds living in their vicinity.

What Does RF/MW Research Show?

Since, as one scientist put it, the only location that is currently free of RF/MW is the back side of the moon, it is no longer possible to do population studies to determine whether exposure to RF/MW causes an increase in certain diseases. If there is no safe level of RF/MW exposure, we cannot rely upon studies that use various exposure levels to demonstrate an adverse response. We can only look back at studies performed or data collected prior to the advent of the ubiquitous FM and microwave radiation of our planet.

One of the factors affecting the outcome of so-called scientific studies is investigator bias. I know of no better example of this than that shown in analyses of childhood cancer statistics surrounding the Sutro tower in San Francisco.

The Sutro tower broadcasts radio and television signals to the San Francisco Bay area. Data on childhood cancer within a seven mile radius of the tower was collected between 1973 and 1988. Two separate analyses of the data have been published.

In 1993, statisticians at the University of California at Berkeley reported their analysis of the Sutro Tower data.[73] They concluded, "the patterns of the major childhood cancers are essentially random with respect to the point source." In other words, they found no correlation between the location of a child's home relative to the tower and the chance of the child developing cancer. The Berkeley article was published in the journal *Social Science Medicine* and is contained in the National Library of Medicine database.

In 2000, Dr. Neil Cherry, a pioneer in researching the effects of electromagnetic fields on human health, reanalyzed the data.[74] Dr. Cherry, an independent researcher with no ties to the broadcasting industry, found not only a significant, not simply a highly significant, but an *extremely significant* increase in the incidence of all cancers in white children living within a seven mile radius of the Sutro tower.

One of the analyses performed by Dr. Cherry compared the incidence of childhood cancer with the child's exposure to radio/television wave radiation. Since waves have a peak and a trough, individual houses receive either a high or low level of exposure. Dr. Cherry's analysis showed a jump in cancer incidence in those houses hit by the peaks of the waves as they moved away from the tower.

Because Dr. Cherry's work was performed and published in New Zealand, where he was Associate Professor of Environmental Health at Lincoln University, it has been almost universally overlooked in the United States. Nevertheless, Dr. Cherry was arguably the world's foremost expert on electromagnetic radiation and human health. His strong background in physics, biophysics, meteorology, and environmental epidemiology made him uniquely suited to evaluate the impact of RF/MW radiation. In 2002, Dr. Cherry was awarded the Royal Honour of Officer of New Zealand Order of Merit for his services to science, education, and community, including his research and teaching work on environmental epidemiology and the health effects of electromagnetic radiation.

Others have found similar increases in cancer surrounding RF/MW antennas. Data collected between 1974 and 1986 confirmed a suspected increase in adult leukemia cases surrounding the Sutton Coldfield television and FM radio transmitter in West Highlands, England.[75] The incidence of skin cancer and bladder cancer was also shown to be higher in locations nearer to the tower. Data collected from 1972 to 1990 in North Sydney, Australia showed that children living near TV towers were almost twice as likely to die of leukemia as children at more distant locations.[76] An analysis of data from an area surrounding a transmitter in Rome, Italy produced a similar result.[77]

Even more telling is the research of Orjan Hallberg and Olle Johansson of the Karolinska Institute in Stockholm, Sweden. Hallberg and Johansson have published several papers looking at disease incidence before and after the introduction of FM radio broadcasting. As is typical of research that is critical to RF/MW technology, their work has been published in small journals such as the *ACNEM Journal*, which is published by the Australian college of Nutrition and Environmental Medicine. Because these publications are not included in the United States' National Library of Medicine database, few people are aware of their findings.

Dr. Johansson, a dermatologist, was intrigued by the sharp rise in malignant melanoma incidence, which began in the mid-twentieth century. While experts espoused the theory that the increase was due to greater sun exposure, Johansson was skeptical. He and Hallberg examined the correlation between melanoma and increased sun exposure of the Swedish population.[78] They were able to do this because residents of Sweden must travel to the beaches of Southern Europe to swim and sunbathe. The availability to do so was limited until charter air flights became available in the 1960s. Hallberg and Johansson found that the number of melanoma deaths and new diagnoses of the disease began to rise well before Swedes began traveling to sunny climes.

Having failed to find a correlation between increased sun exposure and malignant melanoma, they looked for other possible explanations. They discovered that the death rate and incidence of the disease rose in concert with the rise in FM broadcasting in Sweden, suggesting that exposure to radio waves adversely affected the body's ability to respond to and repair damaged cells. New cases began to be diagnosed several years later, suggesting that the FM waves not only impaired the body's response to the cancer, but caused damage that predisposed to the development of the disease.

Having demonstrated a strong correlation between melanoma and FM broadcasts in Sweden, they looked at the relationship between FM broadcasting and malignant melanoma in other countries. They found the same correlation.

One of the observations that caused Johansson to question the theory that malignant melanomas are caused by sun exposure is the fact that they occur most commonly on the trunk of the body, which typically has less sun exposure than the face, neck, and the extremities. This phenomenon has baffled physicians ever since the sun exposure theory was first proposed. Some have even suggested that occasional exposure of one's skin to the sun is more likely to trigger a melanoma than frequent sun exposure. Hallberg and Johansson compared the distribution of malignant melanoma lesions on the body to the strength of the electric current generated in the body by FM radio waves. They discovered that the distribution of melanoma and the distribution of the FM current are a perfect match.

In 2002, Hallberg and Johansson released a study titled "Cancer Trends During the 20th Century."[79] In the paper, they show that mortality rates for bladder, prostate, colon, breast, and lung cancers in the United States, Sweden, and other countries closely parallel that of malignant melanoma. They further demonstrate that these cancers have increased and decreased depending upon the amount of exposure to radio waves during the past hundred years. When FM broadcasting increased in a given location, so did cancer rates. In contrast, when radio broadcasting decreased, so did the incidence of cancer. Incredibly, they found that exposure to radio waves was as significant a factor in the development of lung cancer as cigarette smoking!

Given the correlations between FM broadcasting and cancer, it is alarming to consider a study done in Salzburg, Austria. It found that the RF/MW radiation levels had increased over one hundredfold following the installation of a cellular communication network.[80]

When short-term studies failed to show an increased risk of brain tumors with mobile phone use, representatives of wireless industries, medical organizations, and governmental agencies were quick to proclaim that the devices were safe. Unfortunately, time is not proving that stance to be correct. Two studies released in 2006 showed a significant increase in tumors related to cell phone use. The first showed an increase in non-malignant tumors of the nerve that carries sounds from the ear to the brain (acoustic neuromas) on the side used to listen to the phone.[81] The second showed an increase in gliomas, a type of brain cancer.[82] In both instances, the rise in tumor incidence did not appear until individuals had been using a cellular telephone for ten years.

In 2010, partial results of the World Health Organization sponsored Interphone study were released and heralded as proving that cell phone use does not increase the risk of brain tumors. What the study actually showed is that lifetime exposure to cellular phone frequencies is cumulative and that increased tumor incidence is seen after 1640 lifetime hours of exposure.

As striking as the statistical correlations are (well outside the realm of chance), it is important to determine whether a mechanism exists by which RF/MW radiation could trigger the appearance of cancer in the human body. Research has demonstrated that a mechanism does exist.

In 1995, a landmark study conducted by Doctors Henry Lai and N. P. Singh at the University of Washington's Center for Bioengineering demonstrated that a single two-hour exposure to microwave radiation lower than the government's "safe" level caused breaks in DNA.[83] This was highly significant, since DNA damage is one of the primary triggers for cancer development. Unfortunately, Lai and Singh could not obtain funding to pursue their research into RF/MW effects on DNA.

Following the publication of Lai and Singh's findings, another researcher, Dr. Jerry Phillips, was given a grant by Motorola to perform another experiment on the effects of cellular telephone radiation on animals. Dr. Phillips agreed.

It is important to understand that Dr. Singh is one of the world's leading experts in detection of DNA damage. He developed a technique known as the "comet assay" to identify breaks in DNA strands. His assay has been used to show DNA damage in a wide range of conditions including exposure to chemicals and high frequency radiation. In preparation for his research, Dr. Phillips sent two assistants to Washington to learn how to perform Dr. Singh's comet assay. Only after duplicating Singh's results in other areas did Phillips conduct his experiment on microwave exposure and DNA damage.

Dr. Phillips's results were consistent with those of Lai and Singh.[84] Motorola executives encouraged Phillips to hold off on publishing his data, but he refused.[85] He was unable to obtain funding for further research. Other laboratories subsequently reported that microwave radiation did not cause DNA damage, but they did not use Dr. Singh's sensitive comet assay technology.

Finally, in 2004, twelve research institutions located in seven European countries reported that they had proven conclusively that low level exposure to RF/MW radiation causes genetic damage.[86] Known as the REFLEX study, DNA damage and a change in the action of numerous genes and proteins were shown to occur with great certainty. While their work was done on living cells in the laboratory, it has great implications on what might be expected to occur when whole organisms are exposed to RF/MV radiation. In September 2005, Dr. Zhengping Xu of the Zhejiang University School of Medicine reported that his laboratory had also found a significant increase in DNA damage in cells exposed to RF/MW radiation.[87]

Does RF/MW Radiation Pose a Risk to Human Health?

Dr. Leif Salford, who has spent over fifteen years researching the effect of RF/MW radiation on the brain, has called the expansion of cell phone technology "the world's largest human biological experiment." While no one can authoritatively say how the experiment will turn out, it is clear that there is great cause for concern.

The prevailing attitude in the United States is that RF/MW radiation poses no risk to human health, but increasing numbers of scientists disagree. In 1998, a group of scientists adopted the Vienna Resolution, which stated in part, "biological effects from low intensity [RFR] exposures are scientifically established."[88] The Salzburg resolution of 2000 stated that there is no safe exposure level for RF/MW radiation.[89] The Stewart report that same year urged the United Kingdom to use caution in expansion of wireless technologies until more scientific evidence was available.[90] The Catania Resolution of 2002 also urged caution.[91]

In 2005, the United Kingdom National Radiation Protection Board issued a warning that no child under the age of 8 should use a cell phone.[92] The report also listed concerns about the location of cellular telephone towers. In September 2006, the International Commission for Electromagnetic Safety (ICEMS) released the Benevento Resolution, which stated that the accumulated evidence points to "adverse health effects from occupational and public exposures to electric, magnetic and electromagnetic fields (EMF) at current exposure levels."[93] It was signed by thirty-one leading environmental health scientists from around the world.

Organizations producing materials for the general public have unfortunately been reluctant to include any warnings about the potential dangers of RF/MW radiation. I was therefore encouraged to read the following statement on page seven of the Breast Cancer Fund's 2006 booklet, *State of the Evidence*: "A growing body of evidence implicates nonionizing radiation (electromagnetic fields and radio-frequency radiation [EMF]) as possible contributors to the development of breast cancer. The International Agency for Research on Cancer (IARC) has classified EMF as a possible human carcinogen. Microwaves, radio waves, radar and lights are examples of nonionizing radiation. Everyone in the industrialized world is exposed to electromagnetic fields every day."[94]

Sources of RF/MW Radiation

As I study sources of radio frequency microwave radiation (RF/MW) and the effects of RF/MW on the human body, I am struck with the realization that I am just seeing the tip of the iceberg. What little concern is present about the hazards of RF/MW exposure centers around the use of cellular telephones, but other applications of RF/MW technology are appearing at an astounding rate.

RF/MW radiation is ubiquitous in our environment, meaning that it is present everywhere. Radio, television, and cellular telephone towers are visible evidence that waves are being beamed toward us, but we are also being radiated by satellite radio beams, satellite television waves, and Wi-Fi in an increasing number of public and private establishments; WI-MAX has the ability to provide connectivity within a thirty mile radius, and everyone within its range is continually exposed to microwave radiation. An increasing number of retail items are being labeled with radiofrequency identification (RFID) transponders that are capable of transmitting their signals toward the bodies of consumers who are completely unaware of their presence.

RFID Ink, which can be applied as either a visible or invisible tattoo, is now in use in animals and is being considered for application to military personnel. Can promotion of its use to the civilian population be far behind? After all, a driver's license can be forged and credit cards stolen, but a tattoo is forever.

People who express a concern about cellular telephone towers or power lines often fail to recognize threats that are closer to home. Cordless telephones with base units, cordless headsets, remote control devices, and in-home or office wireless computer networks all radiate RF/MW energy.

We have become so accustomed to these devices that the level of energy they transmit is taken for granted. I gained a sense of their impact when I read a statement by an astronomer. Had Neil Armstrong taken a cell phone to the moon, he suggested, it would have been recognized as the third most powerful source of electromagnetic radiation in the universe, behind only the sun and the Milky Way.

RF/MW Radiation and the Human Nervous System

Earlier in this chapter I reported studies that demonstrate a link between RF/MW radiation and cancer. I also explained what is known about the mechanisms by which such radiation triggers tumor growth. I will now discuss the effects of RF/MW on the neuromuscular system.

Diseases of the nervous system are on the rise, as are diseases involving the muscles. The incidence of Alzheimer's disease in Los Angeles County has been reported to have increased by 250 percent in the past decade. Fibromyalgia, virtually unknown in the early 1970s, is now commonplace. The same is true of attention deficit hyperactivity disorder.

A 2003 review of the medical literature found that in nine of ten published studies the risk of amyotrophic lateral sclerosis (Lou Gehrig's disease) was increased in men who had occupational exposure to electromagnetic fields.[95] Swedish studies showing that men with occupational exposure to electromagnetic fields are 2.3 times more likely to develop Alzheimer's disease and 1.5 times more likely to present with Parkinson's disease strongly suggest that RF/MW exposure is playing a role in the increasing incidence of degenerative nervous system diseases.[96,97]

That RF/MW radiation affects brain and nervous system function has been demonstrated in numerous studies. Many have reported on changes in brain wave patterns (EEG) with exposure to RF/MW. This is not surprising, as brain waves represent electrical activity within the brain. No one questions the fact that cellular telephones interfere with the normal operation of electronic appliances. Airplane passengers are not allowed to use their cell phones from the time the plane is ready for departure to when it has safely landed and is taxiing to the gate. Cellular phone usage is discouraged or banned in hospital intensive care units because of interference with pacemakers, defibrillators, and other electronic devices.

If RF/MW radiation interferes with the normal operation of aircraft guidance systems and other electronic devices, it is logical that it would also interfere with the normal electrical systems within the human body. Evidence now exists that suggests the body is designed to use its own microwaves for intercellular communication. The extremely low strength of the body's signals can easily be disrupted or overridden by today's RF/MW devices. The changes observed following exposure to RF/MW have been found to occur more quickly and be more pronounced in children.

An interesting finding in RF/MW-EEG studies is that the effects are variable. Some individuals are much more sensitive to RF/MW exposure than others. It also appears that individual sensitivity may vary, with a significant effect appearing at some times and not others. This means that when the average reactivity of a group is reported, the actual effect of RF/MW can appear to be much lower than it actually is. (The lack of effect in non-sensitive individuals will dilute the significance of the effect seen in sensitive subjects.)

At least three RF/MW effects provide plausible explanations for how exposure could increase the risk and accelerate the progression of neuromuscular diseases. The first is the adverse effect of RF/MW radiation on what is known as the blood-brain barrier.

The blood-brain barrier is a wonderful example of how intricately the human body is designed. The tiniest blood vessels in the body are called capillaries. Most capillaries are so small that their diameter is just slightly larger than that of a red blood cell. This facilitates the exchange of oxygen between the red blood cells and the tissues through which the blood is flowing. It is also at the capillary level that exchange of nutrients takes place.

Most capillaries of the body allow a relatively free exchange of substances between the blood and the tissues on the other side of the capillary wall. Capillaries in the brain, however, are much more selective. These vessels contain a specialized system of cells lining their walls that protect the brain from potentially harmful substances in the bloodstream while allowing the passage of nutrients required for proper brain function. This system, which involves both physical (tight seams between the cells) and chemical (enzyme) safeguards, is referred to as the blood-brain barrier (BBB).

Studies have demonstrated that RF/MW radiation breaks down the blood-brain barrier. This destroys the body's ability to protect the sensitive tissues of the brain from harmful substances. BBB dysfunction is considered a key component in the process that leads to diseases of the central nervous system, including diseases such as Alzheimer's disease and Parkinson's disease.

A team in the Department of Neurology at Lund University in Lund, Sweden, has done pioneering research in the area of RF/MW damage to the BBB.[98] They first demonstrated that exposure to RF/MW caused the leakage of albumen (a protein) from the bloodstream into the brain. They continued their investigations and subsequently found that the leakage of albumen led to nerve cell damage in multiple areas of the brain (the cortex, the hippocampus, and the basal ganglia).[99]

The lead researcher of the Lund University team is Dr. Leif Salford, a neurosurgeon. He is the individual who first referred to the use of handheld cellular telephones as "the largest human biological experiment ever." He believes that today's generation of cell-phone-using teenagers may suffer from mental deficits or Alzheimer's disease by the time they reach middle age.

The effect of RF/MW radiation on the blood-brain barrier provides one possible explanation for the appearance of what is referred to as "Gulf War Syndrome." Following Operation Desert Storm, many war veterans began to complain of a cluster of symptoms that were not consistent with any known disease. The symptoms included aching muscles, irritability, thick saliva, weight loss, skin rashes, memory loss, chronic fevers, labored breathing, and headaches. Skeptics were quick to suggest that the symptoms were due to a form of mass hysteria, a stress reaction, or were due to any number of diseases that would have occurred in the men and women had they not served in Kuwait. At this point, however, over ten thousand Gulf War veterans have requested examinations because they believe that they are suffering from the syndrome. Their symptoms should not be casually dismissed as imaginary or coincidental.

Many soldiers were exposed to intense RF/MW radiation during the war. This came from various high-tech instruments, thousands of radio communication devices, and widespread radar use. Pesticides, including DDT, malathion, fenitrorthion, propuxur, deltamethrin, and permethrin, were reportedly used extensively during the war. Destruction of Iraqi weapons stores is known to have released nerve agents including sarin and cyclosarin into the environment.

While the connection cannot be proven at this late date, what is now known about the effect of RF/MW on the blood-brain barrier suggests that the risk of exposure to toxic chemicals would have been much greater than normally expected. The level of toxins leaking into the central nervous systems of soldiers would have been significantly higher than from exposures to the chemicals outside of a high RF/MW environment. The effects of such exposure would likewise exceed those predicted based upon exposures in low RF/MW settings.

A frightening aspect of the research into the breakdown of the BBB by RF/MW is that some scientists believe that the loss of the BBB is irreversible. I am cautiously optimistic that is not the case, but unless the association between RF/MW exposure and increased toxicity from exposure to chemicals is disproved, it would be wise for individuals to use maximum precautions such as protective gloves and masks when working with chemicals in yards, gardens, and around the home.

The second way in which RF/MW can adversely affect neuromuscular function is by causing damage to proteins. Researchers in Helsinki, Finland have shown that proteins are altered by RF/MW exposure and how those changes in protein expression can adversely impact cell function.[100] Italian scientists have demonstrated that RF/MW radiation damages myoglobin, the chief oxygen-carrying protein in muscle tissue.[101] Loss of myoglobin functionality would be expected to result in a decreased efficiency of muscle activity.

Free radical damage is believed to be one of the leading causes of aging and disease development. One of the avenues of treatment for Alzheimer's disease and Parkinson's disease is the use of drugs to slow oxidative damage in the brain. RF/MW radiation has also been shown to increase oxidative damage in tissues.

Interestingly, extracts of ginkgo biloba, a tree that is resistant to damage from short wave radiation (nuclear radiation), have been shown to reduce mobile phone-induced oxidative stress in the brain.[102] This implies that while RF/MW can cause adverse chemical activity (increased oxidative damage), substances that protect against oxidative damage from chemical agents can also protect against oxidative damage from electromagnetic stress.

The fourth way in which RF/MW radiation may cause neuromuscular disease is by diminishing the ability of a chemical, acetylcholine, to transmit messages from cell to cell. Scientists at the University of Rome have shown that exposure to RF/MW decreases the ability of acetylcholine to transmit signals.[103] Several drugs that are designed to increase acetylcholine activity in the brain have been introduced in recent years for the treatment of degenerative diseases such as Alzheimer's.

Other studies have focused not on the mechanisms by which RF/MW can adversely affect muscles and nerves, but upon the actual effects of RF/MW observed in exposed individuals. I discussed the challenges involved in observational studies at length earlier this chapter. The primary challenge is that at this point in time everyone is exposed to high level RF/MW radiation, making studies comparing an exposed group to an unexposed group impossible. The only thing that can be compared is temporary intensity of exposure, which often yields highly variable results. A second difficulty is that effects of exposure may not appear for a decade or more, making short-term studies relatively meaningless. Finally, the bias of industry-funded studies makes an honest analysis of the effects of RF/MW radiation difficult, if not impossible.

Nevertheless, a few studies are worthy of mention. In 1989, medical researchers at Zhejiang Medical University in the People's Republic of China, which did not have as extensive coverage of RF/MW towers as the United States and Europe, found that people who lived or worked near radio towers or radar installations had slower reaction times and poorer short-term memory than those not living or working in close proximity to RF/MW systems.[104]

In 1996, the Latvian Academy of Sciences reported that school children living in the area of the Skrunda Radio Location Station in Latvia had less developed memory and attention, slower reaction times, and diminished neuromuscular endurance.[105] I believe the experiment was able to show a difference because Latvia did not have the number of wave-generating towers found in Western Europe.

RF Syndrome

Apart from the effects documented in scientific studies, a syndrome has emerged. It is called by various names, including electromagnetic sensitivity syndrome, microwave sickness, radio wave sickness or RF syndrome. Commonly reported symptoms include insomnia, dizziness, nausea, headaches, fatigue, memory loss, inability to concentrate, depression, chest discomfort, and ringing in the ears. While the existence of the phenomenon is questioned by skeptics, studies have shown that some individuals are, indeed, hypersensitive to electromagnetic radiation.

While the syndrome is presenting in ever-increasing numbers of people, it is not new. Dr. Arthur Firstenberg, a leading expert in RF/MW-induced disease, reports that it first appeared among employees who worked with radar equipment in the 1950s and 1960s. It was also reported by operators of industrial microwave heaters and sealers. With the expansion of RF/MW technologies, what was once an occupational disease from which individuals could find relief by changing jobs has become a universal challenge from which there is no escape. Dr. Firstenberg estimates that as much as a third of the population is already affected to some degree.[106]

French researchers with the National Institute of Applied Sciences surveyed 530 people, half of whom lived within three hundred meters (slightly more than the length of three football fields) of a cellular telephone tower.[107] They found a significant increase in tiredness, headache, sleep disturbance, irritability, depression, loss of memory, dizziness, loss of sex drive, nausea, loss of appetite, and visual disturbances. Those symptoms correlate strongly with those reported by individuals who suffer from RF syndrome.

Subsequently, a similar survey was carried out in Murcia, Spain.[108] The investigators measured the microwave power density in the homes of those surveyed and found a significant correlation between the severity of the symptoms reported and the strength of the microwave radiation within the home. The severity of the symptoms reported increased as the level of exposure increased.

Individuals who experience microwave sickness typically find that their complaints fall upon deaf ears. The highest-profile individual to report electromagnetic sensitivity is Gro Harlem Brundtland, who in 2002, while head of the World Health Organization, told a Norwegian journalist that cell phones were banned from her office in Geneva because she personally becomes ill if she comes within four meters (approximately thirteen feet) of one.[109] Dr. Brundtland is also a former Prime Minister of Norway and is a medical doctor. She was publicly ridiculed for making the statement. She stepped down from her position after just one term.

It is time that individuals who are experiencing microwave sickness be taken seriously. The person who today arrogantly refers to the disease as "psychosomatic" or an exaggerated response to stress just may be on the other side of the fence tomorrow. Our ability as a society to ignore the relentless march of RF/MW-related illness reminds me of the words of Martin Niemoeller, a Christian who resisted Adolph Hitler's takeover of the church in Germany and, as a result, spent many years in a concentration camp:

First they came for the communists, and I did not speak out—
because I was not a communist;
Then they came for the socialists, and I did not speak out—
because I was not a socialist;
Then they came for the trade unionists, and I did not speak out—
because I was not a trade unionist;
Then they came for the Jews, and I did not speak out—
because I was not a Jew;
Then they came for me—
and there was no one left to speak out for me.

Who will be left to speak out when the rate of cancer is two per person and Alzheimer's disease affects a majority of those who should be in the prime of their life? Will it matter? I have adapted Niemoeller's words to our generation:

ADHD appeared, and I was not concerned—
because my child did not have ADHD;
Fibromyalgia emerged, and I was not concerned—
because I did not have fibromyalgia;

107

Cancer incidence rose, and I was not concerned—
  because I did not have cancer;
People reported RF sensitivity, and I was not concerned—
  because RF did not bother me;
Now I am sick—
  and there is no one left to be concerned for me.

Protective Devices

Having outlined the dangers of radiofrequency/microwave radiation (RF/MW), I feel compelled to make a confession. Despite what I feel to be clear and indisputable evidence that RF/MW exposure has a profoundly adverse effect upon human health, I am hopelessly addicted to RF/MW conveniences. True, my wife and I have not owned a microwave oven for many years, but we are not technophobes.

I am not willing to give up my computer and its word processing capabilities for a manual Smith-Corona typewriter. I value the freedom of movement that is provided by portable and cellular phone technology. I still remember the confinement imposed by being "on call" for my medical practice prior to the advent of cellular technology. The importance of attending any function or leaving my home for any other reason was always weighed against the anxiety that resulted from being "paged" (by radio frequency) and needing to quickly find a public telephone.

I have a wireless computer network in my home, I have a "Pike Pass" in my car that allows me to bypass toll booths on Oklahoma's turnpikes, and I occasionally watch television or listen to FM radio stations. I use remote control devices to change television channels and to unlock my car. A wireless doorbell alerts me to the arrival of visitors.

No, I am not willing to give up the convenience provided by RF/MW technologies. Even if I were, it would be an exercise in futility. It is impossible to escape RF/MW radiation today. If I did not own a computer, I would still be exposed to wireless networks as I enter stores, restaurants, and hotels. If I threw away my cell phone, I would still be bombarded by the microwaves seeking the hundreds of thousands of other cell phones in use. If I were to rid my home of radios and had no television, I would continue to be hit by television and FM waves beamed from broadcast antennas or satellites.

You and I cannot flee from RF/MW radiation. The earth is blanketed by it. I recently traveled to remote areas of the Rocky Mountains and never lost the signal from XM Satellite Radio. The nearest location to be relatively free of RF/MW radiation is said to be the back side of the moon, which I understand is quite inhospitable. That being the case, what are we to do?

I predict that if humankind survives, historians will not condemn our generation for pursuing and utilizing RF/MW technology, but rather for discouraging research into the effects associated with its use. They will be disheartened that the findings of studies demonstrating potential dangers to human health were suppressed. They will not condemn the research that led to the development of RF/MW devices, but they will disparage the time when RF/MW-sensitive individuals were dismissed as hysterical or said to be imagining their symptoms.

I do not believe that history will look kindly upon those who disparaged researchers seeking effective ways of protecting the human body from RF/MW radiation, calling them pseudoscientists, quacks, charlatans, or frauds. I am quite certain that future generations will marvel that RF/MW protection was labeled a scam by those who refused to acknowledge the dangers inherent in low-frequency radiation. They will be astounded that people were warned against wasting money on devices designed to provide protection from RF/MW exposure.

The first energetic protection devices that came to my attention were those developed by a German inventor named Manfred Bauer. Mr. Bauer had become interested in energetic devices after he developed cancer. When his physicians could not tell him *why* the cancer had occurred, he began asking others. An elderly natural healer told him that it was because he was sleeping in an area of low electromagnetic energy. He investigated and found that his bed was, indeed, located in an area of low energy. Other cancer patients he met while receiving radiation treatments asked him to check their homes and he found that every one of them had been sleeping in a low energy zone.

Manfred Bauer was not the first to discover this phenomenon. In 1929, a German scientist, Gustav Freiherr von Pohl, mapped the course of underground streams beneath Vilsbiburg, Germany.[110] (Moving water disrupts the energy field generated by the earth's magnetic core.) He then compared the registry of individuals who had died from cancer with his map. He found that all forty-eight people who had died of cancer in Vilsbiburg had been sleeping directly above one of the underground streams.

In 1976, an Austrian teacher, Kathe Bachler, published her findings regarding electromagnetic energy levels and school performance. She reported that 95 percent of "problem children" slept in beds or sat in desks located in a danger zone. She subsequently examined five hundred cancer deaths and discovered that in every instance the individual had been sleeping in an area of low energy.[111]

After learning of the link between underground streams and cancer development, Manfred Bauer moved his bed. He continued conventional therapy and successfully recovered from his cancer. Having done so, he set about to find a way to improve energy levels in the environment. He observed that rain water is naturally high in energy. (This explains why a lawn that is barely surviving with water from a sprinkling system will immediately turn a deeper green and begin to grow more quickly following a thunderstorm.)

Manfred learned that it was the rising and falling, and warming and cooling of the water droplets in clouds that generated the energy. His greatest challenge was finding a way to stabilize the captured energy and prevent it from dissipating. Having successfully devised a means of taking water to a stable higher energy level, he began manufacturing devices that could transmit that energy to the surrounding space and to other objects. He developed appliances that were capable of increasing the level of energy over a variety of distances. Some devices would enhance the energy level within a two foot radius, while others could increase the energy level within a fifty foot radius.

Mr. Bauer's devices were effective—I still have one in my home—but there were challenges associated with their use. One was that while the energized water was sealed within plastic containers, the water would often slowly evaporate. Another was that if one of the devices was exposed to x-ray, as might occur during shipping or in an airport, its energy would be lost. The same would happen if it was exposed to microwaves. If one of the appliances was inadvertently placed near a cellular telephone or a microwave oven, its effectiveness would be lost.

Soon after Manfred Bauer's water-based devices were introduced, other RF/MW protective appliances began to appear. I have evaluated most of these, and have my personal favorites. I will explain why this is so. Bear in mind, however, that RF/MW protection is evolving. None of the available appliances have been submitted to the level of scrutiny demanded by their skeptics, but that does not mean that they are not based upon sound scientific principles. While none of them have been in use for the number of decades necessary to prove their long-term effectiveness, immediate improvements in muscle strength during exposures to microwaves or electromagnetic fields can be demonstrated.

I do not pretend to understand the intricate details on how the devices are constructed or how they function. I have a basic understanding of the theories upon which they are based, but I am not an expert in quantum physics, spin theory, string theory, and zero point energy. I know that the science of nanotechnology exists, but I know very little about its substance.

Bear with me, and don't panic if you feel a bit lost during the next two paragraphs. I will come back to practicality immediately.

Simply stated, quantum physics deals with sub-atomic particles and their energies. Spin theory states that electron-spin speed and direction is critical to maintaining stability of matter in our universe. String theory is an attempt to unify basic laws that govern the physical universe, including the law of gravity and the laws of electricity and magnetism. String theory states that all matter is made up of vibrating strings, and that the state of matter is determined to a large extent by the intrinsic vibrational frequencies of an object and how those vibrations respond to external forces. Zero point energy refers to the lowest energy state of any substance.

Nanotechnologies deal with applications on the atomic level. One nanometer is one-billionth of a meter. The distance between atoms in a molecule, for example, is measured in nanometers. Nanoenergies are similarly small. For example, a tesla is the scientific unit used to measure the strength of a magnetic field. One nanotesla is one-billionth of a tesla.

What that means, in practical terms, is that the human body, like all material objects, has basic vibrational frequencies. When those vibrational frequencies are disrupted by external forces, including RF/MW radiation, disease is likely to develop. Devices that act to shield those vibrations from external forces should be capable of preventing the development of disease.

The most widely recognized RF/MW protective device is the Q–Link. Its popularity is due in large part to the promotional efforts of popular speakers and celebrities such as Tony Robbins. The Q-Link is composed of a resonating cell and an amplifying coil. The resonating cell contains crystalline elements that pick up the subtle vibrations of the human body, which are then amplified by the coil to provide a cocoon of protection from external energy sources.

The Q-Link does provide a level of protection from external radiation. The reason I have not chosen to personally use a Q-Link and why I do not recommend it as the best device for this purpose is that it selectively tunes to the energies of the person who is wearing it. The Q-Link manufacturer specifically advises against sharing a Q-Link with anyone but the original wearer because it becomes tuned to that individual's specific frequencies.

While many view the "personalization" feature of the Q-Link as an advantage, I do not. When the human body becomes diseased, its vibratory pattern changes. Homeopathy is a system of medicine that uses the intrinsic vibratory frequencies of substances to correct abnormal vibratory patterns in disease and restore health. This being the case, if an individual is in perfect health when he or she begins wearing a Q-Link it should work beautifully to maintain health. On the other hand, if a disease state is developing it would appear that a Q-Link would tune to that vibration and tend to maintain the disease state, rather than promote a return to a normal state of health.

My reasoning is based upon experience with foot problems. For a number of years, I referred individuals who presented with plantar faschiitis or similar foot disorders to a podiatrist who would take imprints of the person's feet and provide a custom-made orthotic (support). Then I ran across a study that showed that people who bought standard over-the-counter orthotics fared better than those who obtained the personalized supports.[112] At first I was puzzled, because the findings ran counter to what I would have predicted. Upon reflection, however, the findings made perfect sense. The standard orthotics were encouraging an abnormal foot to mold to the shape of a healthy foot while the custom-made devices were simply maintaining the abnormal shape and attempting to prevent further deterioration.

Another popular device is the bioelectric shield. The bioelectric shield, like the Q-Link, makes use of natural crystalline elements, which are encased in a sterling silver case. Like the Q-Link, the bioelectric shield conforms to an individual's body frequencies. The manufacture advises against letting anyone but the original wearer use the device, stating that the appliance may make another person feel uncomfortable if the individual frequencies are different.

The Bioshield is said to have been charged in a special room during the manufacturing process. The wearer is advised to recharge the device by hanging it in daylight for at least six hours each month and to avoid exposure to moonlight, which is said to drain the Bioshield's protective energy. While I have seen no data suggesting that the Bioshield is adversely affected by exposure to different types of radiation, its tendency to recharge or discharge depending upon the type of light exposure makes me wary of its long-range ability to maintain an optimum energetic field.

My personal preference is to use devices that, like the standard orthotics, are manufactured to shield the body from chaotic vibratory frequencies or, when possible, augment and amplify frequencies known to be consistent with optimum physical health. This is possible because of the pioneering work of Nobel Prize winning physicists William Bragg, Sr. and William Bragg, Jr. The Braggs were awarded the Nobel Prize in 1915 for the development of a formula that describes the effect of crystal spacing on electromagnetic energy frequencies. By using what is now known as Bragg's law, manufacturers can effectively produce devices that affect energies reaching the body down to the nanotesla range. These devices are manufactured by creating a silicon matrix that selectively amplifies the frequencies of the earth's electromagnetic field that are conducive to human health while either blocking or redirecting chaotic energies that disrupt the normal function of the body. Silicon matrix appliances are not affected by the body's intrinsic vibratory pattern, but rather encourage the pattern to return to that known to be consistent with optimum health. Unlike the water-based appliances, they are not damaged by exposure to x-rays or microwaves and, since they are solid glass, there is no risk of failure due to evaporation.

I have used and recommended matrix appliances for many years. A basic device is an E-Crystal, which effectively shields the body from external energy sources. It creates a cocoon of protection approximately three feet in diameter. Therefore carrying the device in a shirt pocket or wearing it as a necklace provides the greatest total body protection. Carrying the appliance in a pants pocket will provide protection, but the brain may not be fully protected because the head will be located at or beyond the perimeter of the circle of protection. The appliance is still manufactured, but I no longer recommend it because it does not provide the level of protection provided by more technically advanced devices.

A series of matrix devices has been introduced over the years. These include the E-Tag, the QE pendant, and the Q2 pendant. Since their effectiveness has been eclipsed by newer technologies, there is not a need to discuss them in detail. They still provide protection to individuals using them, but I do not consider them devices of choice for those seeking a personal protective device at this time.

The technology I am personally using at the present time is the EP2 Pendant. This device is non-polar, and in addition to shielding the body from chaotic energies and encouraging alignment of cells in the body, the EP2 selectively identifies and amplifies life-supporting frequencies. This technology is a practical application of zero point energy and quantum energy theory.

Simply stated, an access "door" or "gateway" is placed in the device that allows the sorting of energies with a positive counter-clockwise electron spin from those with a body energy-depleting clockwise electron spin. The sorted energies are then amplified through "light" angles, creating an intense field of these organized life-supporting energies. Any chaos that then enters this field is immediately organized. The device itself has absolutely nothing to do with the effect. It simply holds the technology that has been mechanically placed, from a quantum perspective, into its silicone-like structure.

These are the major devices available for personal protection from RF/MW radiation that I am aware of at this time. I have no doubt that additional devices will be introduced in the future. Other devices are available that are not worn on the body, but are attached to a phone or computer, placed in a room or used in a home to provide localized protection.

I am often asked, "Where are the studies that prove that energetic protective appliances are effective?" This is because physicians and the public at large have been conditioned to believe that the only acceptable evidence of effectiveness of a medical product or device is what is referred to as a placebo-controlled, double-blinded, crossover study. Placebo-controlled means that one group receives an active device and a second group a device that looks like the active one, but which is actually inactive. Double-blinded means that neither the study subjects nor those conducting the research know which products or devices are active and which are inactive. Crossover means that after a period of time those subjects that originally received an active device are given an inactive one and those who began with an inactive device receive an active product.

At this point there are no double-blinded, placebo-controlled, crossover studies on the effectiveness of electromagnetic protective appliances, nor are there likely to be any in the future. The ability to conduct long-term controlled studies of any kind is extremely limited. The vast majority of medical studies are conducted over a matter of months. Studies that go on for over two years are rare, and studies greater than five years in length are nearly nonexistent. Since studies of cell phone use tend to show an increase in number of tumors only after ten or more years of use, a controlled study involving tens of thousands of people over a period of ten to fifteen years would be required to demonstrate benefit from use of a protective appliance. That, however, would not settle the issue. Researchers would then need to add a "cross-over" element to the study, meaning that the subjects receiving the protective appliance and those using a placebo device would need to be switched and the study repeated. We are now looking at a time frame of two to three decades before a study meeting the standard for scientific proof could be completed.

We live in a world that is still not convinced that RF/MW radiation poses a threat to human health; we live in a society that rejects the results of studies that demonstrate an increased risk of brain tumors from cell phone use. It would be impossible to obtain funding for a study seeking to prove that people can be protected from a danger most authorities do not believe exists. Even if such a study were to be designed and implemented, it would take at least ten to fifteen years to obtain any meaningful results.

Fortunately, it is not necessary to rely solely upon placebo-controlled, double-blinded, crossover studies to determine whether appliances provide a measure of protection from RF/MW radiation. One need only observe their immediate effect upon the human body.

One day I went to a local Radio Shack to purchase some batteries. One of the sales associates approached me. He was at least 6' 2" tall and his physique was that of an avid body builder. Noticing a protective appliance on my cell phone he leaned over and whispered, "You wasted your money; those things don't do anything!"

"Really?" I responded. "Are you willing to let me do a little test?"

"Okay," he replied, hesitantly.

I asked him to hold his right arm steady as I attempted to push it down. Given his strength, I could probably have done a chin-up without the slightest movement of his arm. I then dialed his cell phone number and asked him to once again hold his arm steady as he talked on the phone. I could easily drop his arm using only one finger. I exchanged phones and repeated the arm challenge. His arm was as stable holding my phone with the "worthless" device as it had been when he wasn't holding an active cell phone.

I would like to report that he asked me where to obtain the protective appliance I was using, but he simply handed back my cell phone and walked away shaking his head. Skepticism regarding cell phone risks is so great that many people will not listen to what their own body is telling them. They prefer to explain away the loss of the ability to hold a muscle steady as some sort of parlor trick rather than an actual physical effect upon the body. It is not a trick; the failure of the muscle to lock when challenged is the result of an attack on the body's electromagnetic integrity. Although it is not routinely performed by most physicians, testing a muscle reflex is as valid as testing a knee jerk with a rubber hammer. I will address muscle response testing in more detail in the next chapter.

The physics behind protective appliance technology is as sound as that behind the devices that operate on radio frequencies and microwaves. An immediate effect upon the body's integrity can easily be demonstrated. It is foolhardy and dangerous to refuse to use the appliances that are available until a double-blinded, placebo-controlled, crossover study demonstrates a decrease in the incidence of cancer and diseases of the nervous system with their use.

You may or may not agree with my assessment of the available devices, but I want to be sure that the key point is clearly understood: Non-ionizing radiation is a real and present danger, and the level of individual exposure to RF/MW radiation is increasing rapidly. Shielding devices are available, and while they may prove to be imperfect, they provide the best protection available at this time. Select one and use it consistently. Do what you can to avoid becoming one of the casualties of the world's largest experiment.

Chapter 11
Run a Systems Check

Pleasant words are like a honeycomb, Sweetness to the soul and health to the bones.
– Proverbs 16:24

I once read that the best sermons are those that God first works out in the life of the preacher. The thought resonates with me because so many of the resources I draw upon to help individuals restore and maintain their health were acquired through personal necessity. They were added to my armamentarium because I was facing a health challenge that failed to respond to measures with which I was already familiar.

My Introduction to a Body Computer Check

Such was the case with a technique that runs a check of the body's central computer. Early in 2008, I developed a painful right sacroiliac joint. The cause was not obvious. I suspected I had twisted it while lifting something or carrying a grandchild, but I could not point to a specific event that had triggered the condition. Nutritional supports to help the body clear inflammation failed to resolve the pain. Energy appliances directed to the joint gave minimal relief. The joint felt as though it needed to pop, so I visited a chiropractor friend who is normally able to fix skeletal issues with a simple adjustment. This time his attempt to correct the condition only worsened the pain.

By avoiding lifting, I could keep the pain at a level I could live with. Nevertheless, it was clear that something was wrong. In March, Rosalie and I drove fourteen hours to Atlanta. We were there for only two days before driving fourteen hours back to Oklahoma. Two days after we returned home, we drove ten hours to Austin, Texas. The hours of riding in a car had a profoundly detrimental effect. By the time I arrived in Austin, I could not stand upright because of the pain.

I managed to get through the weekend. On our return trip we stopped in Dallas to pick up some items from one of our suppliers, Fred Van Liew. Fred saw my bent posture and said, "Come here." He touched a few points on my body and tested my muscle response. He tapped out a sequence along my spine, but never touched the troubled sacroiliac joint. Immediately the pain was gone, and I was able to stand and walk normally. The pain has never returned.

I was amazed. It was clear that Fred knew something about assisting the body's healing mechanisms that I did not. It was also clear that I needed to learn the technique.

In August, I returned to Dallas to learn how to run a system check on the body's central computer. Yes, the body has a computer. It controls nearly everything you do. As you are reading this, you are not actively controlling your blood sugar level, your heart rate, your various hormone levels, or any of the nearly infinite number of reactions needed to keep your body working properly. All of those functions are on autopilot, controlled by your body's central computer.

As I began to integrate computer checks into my practice, it quickly became clear that I had discovered another key to the wellness puzzle. People have reported more immediate and lasting results from the technique than any other single strategy I have employed to help them restore their health.

A woman who had been feeling tired for two years despite an excellent nutritional regimen called the day after her visit to report that she felt great. Individuals with a history of severe food allergies have been able to return to a normal diet. Others were able to reduce the amount of medication they had been taking for arthritis pain.

A mother brought in a six-year-old girl who was crying loudly. She could not tell me what had happened, but she could not move her right knee. Within seconds of tapping the appropriate spot, she stopped crying, jumped up, and began playing.

Those are but a few examples. I know there will always be exceptions, but the overwhelming majority of people who allow me to run a computer system check sequence and correct weaknesses as they are found are amazed by how much better they feel at the end of the office visit.

Why Run a Computer Check?

The theory behind talking to the body's computer is quite simple. Computer programmers use languages that allow them to communicate with machines. This allows them to create effective operating systems and an infinite variety of applications on which the machines may be put to work. Contacting specific points on the body will cause a muscle reflex to be less if a particular program is not functioning properly. Identification of these points has allowed practitioners to develop programming languages for the body.

Once a computer program has been written, it should continue to perform the functions for which it was designed. Unfortunately, program files can be damaged, causing the application to operate ineffectively or not at all. Almost everyone who has ever used a computer has experienced the frustration of being unable to access a document or open an application because the file has been corrupted. The most common causes of corruption are said to be bad sectors on storage media, lost clusters, cross-linked files, malfunctioning antivirus software, viruses, and system crashes.

The human body has been programmed to effectively repair itself and maintain optimum health. Unfortunately, just as programs written for machines can become corrupted, so can the programs that manage body processes. Unlike machine programs that generally become completely inoperative when files are damaged, human programs typically continue to operate to varying degrees.

It may not be readily apparent that a particular body program has been corrupted, but the fact that it is not performing optimally will severely compromise the body's ability to maintain itself. Over time, symptoms of disease will appear. Addressing symptoms when they arise may bring temporary relief, but true healing will not take place unless the damaged program is repaired. Running a system check is a means of identifying defective programs within the body and effectively restoring their normal function.

Programming Languages

In researching this subject I discovered that there are thousands of programming languages for interacting with man-made computers. This does not mean that one is right and the others wrong. Someone who is fluent in a particular programming language is able to produce results using it. Results will vary depending upon the sophistication of the language being used and the skill of the person using it.

It is therefore not surprising that a number of systems capable of interacting with the body's central computer have emerged. While most of them were developed in the latter half of the twentieth century, their roots date back to the mapping of the meridian system of energy flow in China over five thousand years ago. Body programming languages may be as simple as applying pressure to a few acupuncture points, or they may involve checking dozens of body points and using sequential maneuvers to correct errors that are detected.

There are many ways the body's computer programs can be damaged. Just as software viruses or power surges can disrupt the smooth operation of programs on a personal computer, viral infections and other physical or emotional stressors can cause glitches in the programs that are designed to keep the systems of the body functioning at peak efficiency. Consequently, directing the body to restore those programs to their original state will have as great an impact on the activity of the body as repairing a defective program will have in the operation of a man-made computer.

Muscle Response Testing

Many techniques use manual muscle testing to communicate with the body. Although some who have not bothered to research the technique suggest that it is some sort of parlor trick being played on gullible subjects, the mechanism of manual muscle testing is closely related to a test most physicians perform in their offices every day.

I have been doing physical examinations for nearly forty years. The aspect of a routine examination that is often most intriguing to the person being examined and any family members who may be present is the elicitation of deep tendon reflexes—the knee jerk for example. Children are particularly amazed when their arm or leg jumps without any conscious effort on their part. Some suggest that I am a magician.

While a reflex response to a tap just below the kneecap may appear magical, it is not. Several reactions occur instantaneously to cause the limb to move. When the tendon is tapped sharply the muscle to which it is attached is stretched. A nerve carries the message that the muscle is being stretched to the spinal cord where it is linked to an outgoing nerve that carries a signal back down to the muscle telling it to contract. Another nerve simultaneously delivers a message to the muscle on the back of the leg telling it to relax. The result is a muscle twitch that causes the arm or leg to jump. A message is also delivered to the brain, reporting that the tendon has been tapped, but by the time a person can consciously react the knee jerk has already occurred.

It is well-documented that stimulation of the skin can trigger reflexes that affect internal organs. For example, if the body is suddenly immersed in cold water the heart rate immediately increases and there is an uncontrolled inspiratory gasp. This gasp reflex is believed to be the cause of death in many kayaking mishaps.

Talking to the body's computer system relies upon a muscle reflex that is linked to the body's autonomic nervous system—the system that automatically controls breathing, heart rate, and other body activities.

The activity of skeletal muscles is mediated by nerve cells that lie in a section of the spinal cord called the anterior horn. Anterior horn nerve cells can be voluntarily activated from the brain, but they are also influenced by information arriving from the skin, joints, tendons, and internal structures of the body.

If all is as it should be, muscles are kept in a state of readiness. When a stimulus—like touching a hot stove—appears, they react instantly. If the anterior horn cells are receiving information that something is amiss with an organ, however, the muscles are not prepared to react reflexively when stimulated. Muscles that are ready to react are said to be "conditionally facilitated" and those that are not are said to be "conditionally inhibited."

If a muscle that is facilitated is challenged, it will respond by locking up to resist the challenge. If the muscle is inhibited, however, it will not react reflexively and the lock will not occur. Therefore, by manually challenging a muscle and feeling for a reflexive lock it is possible to determine whether it is facilitated or inhibited.

Manual muscle testing was introduced by physical therapists Henry and Florence Kendall in 1949. In 1964, Dr. George Goodheart began testing individual muscles using the techniques described by the Kendalls. He soon discovered that he could restore strength to a weak muscle by simply applying pressure to trigger points within the muscle. He subsequently noted relationships between muscle weakness and disease or weakness of internal organs, and he found that by correcting the muscle weakness, he was often able to trigger improvement in the function of the organ that was linked to that muscle.

Some who studied Goodheart's work refined and expanded it. Dr. Victor Frank and Dr. C. Harold Havlic worked closely together to develop a system known as Total Body Modification (TBM). Dr. Robin Hyman has drawn on research from many sources to develop a system called Body Specific Analysis (BSA). In effective systems, the test results are reproducible from practitioner to practitioner and corrective measures are consistently effective in restoring proper function.[113]

Today there are thousands of practitioners who have been trained in various systems of therapeutic touch—languages that talk to the body in much the same way programming languages allow software developers to talk to computers. Restoring the functional activity of body programs is another piece in the wellness puzzle. When the body's internal processes are functioning effectively and efficiently, healing is able to proceed unimpeded. Nutritional supports are utilized more effectively and health challenges resolve more quickly. If you seem to have reached an impasse on your wellness journey, you may find it helpful to visit someone who can talk to your body and restore your central computer to its original settings.

Chapter 12

Deal with Stress Like a Duck Deals with Water

Be anxious for nothing, but in everything by prayer and supplication, with thanksgiving, let your requests be made known to God; and the peace of God, which surpasses all understanding, will guard your hearts and minds through Christ Jesus.
– Philippians 4:6-7

How does a duck deal with water? It swims in it and lets it roll off of its back. Stress is inevitable in life. You're swimming in it most of the time. The key in dealing with stress is developing habits that allow you to let it roll off your back.

The Challenge of Stress

The June 6, 1983, cover story of *Time* magazine was entitled "Stress!" The article called stress "The epidemic of the eighties" and identified stress as the number one health problem in the United States. The situation does not appear to have improved; on the contrary, the number of people affected by stress appears to have increased significantly.

A 1983 survey reported that 55 percent of respondents felt great stress at least once a week. The survey was repeated in 1996. By then 75 percent of those interviewed reported experiencing "great stress" at least once a week. A third said that they felt that way at least twice a week.[114] A 2000 Communications Workers Union survey found that 84 percent of workers felt more stressed at work than five years previously. Only 5 percent of those interviewed did not consider stress to be a problem.[115]

"Do you think it's stress?" I've been asked that question many times over the years. In nearly every instance, the person asking the question was concerned that pressure at home or on the job was responsible for the symptoms that he or she was experiencing at the time. My answer has always been the same: "Stress causes nothing, but aggravates everything."

What Is Stress?

Before discussing stress it is important to define what it is. Stress is simply a challenge given to the adaptive abilities of the body, mind, and spirit. If the body, mind, and spirit are capable of rising to the challenge, stress can carry an individual to new levels of accomplishment. If they are not, and adaptive mechanisms fail, illness will ultimately appear.

Stress can be physical, such as sustaining a burn or undergoing a surgical procedure; mental, as in dealing with a strained relationship or taking on additional responsibilities at work; or spiritual, as in having goals or dreams ridiculed or challenged. Stress can be either beneficial, taking you to new heights, or harmful, resulting in a mental or physical breakdown. It is not so much what happens to you, as how you respond that determines the outcome. The question is not, "Am I stressed?" but rather, "Am I up to the challenge?"

Stress as a Disease Trigger

Stress, no matter how intense or what the source, is incapable of causing any illness of its own accord. Another predisposing factor must be present. For example, if there is no plaque buildup in the coronary arteries, a heart attack will not occur no matter how stressful the situation.

It must also be recognized, however, that stress is often the trigger that accounts for the appearance of a disease and that it contributes greatly to the severity of the symptoms that are present. If plaque is present in the coronary arteries, the body's response to stress may destabilize the condition and trigger a heart attack.

When adaptive mechanisms fail, the breakdown generally appears at the weakest point. If an individual has a predisposition to an ulcer due to the presence of an organism called H-pylori in the stomach, abdominal pain or bleeding may appear. If, on the other hand, an individual has narrowed coronary arteries, he or she may experience chest pain. That is why I say, "Stress causes nothing, but aggravates everything."

In 1967, Dr. Thomas H. Holmes and Dr. Richard H. Rahe of the University of Washington published the results of their work on the relationship between social stress and illness in the *Journal of Psychosomatic Research*.[116] By assigning "Life Change Units" to a number of life events (see Table 1), they were able to predict the likelihood of the appearance of a significant illness or injury in the life of an individual experiencing the events.

They found that someone who accrued more than 300 life change units over a twelve-month period had an 80 percent chance of experiencing a serious illness or injury within the next two years. In contrast, an individual who experienced 150 life change units or less had only a 37 percent chance of developing a serious illness within the same time frame.

While the Holmes/Rahe scale is a general indicator of the effect of various life events on the health of an individual, it is important to recognize that some people are far more resilient than others. One of five individuals with over 300 life change units did not experience any recognizable ill effect from the stress, while a third of those evaluated were affected with fewer than 150 life change units.

Stress Management

Since stress in an inevitable part of life, each of us should seek to become one of those adaptable individuals who continue to do well regardless of external circumstances. One of the keys to successfully managing stress is advance preparation. If our body, soul, and spirit have been given consistent support and nourishment, we will almost certainly be able to withstand the challenges of life. If, however, one or more of these aspects has been neglected, we are likely to fail the test when it comes.

The most important element in stress management is developing and cultivating a relationship with the Creator. That this is possible is one of the greatest mysteries of life. That so many fail to avail themselves of the opportunity is even more bewildering. When that relationship is strong, based upon a moment-by-moment and day-by-day interaction, no amount of stress can quench one's spirit.

Table 1	The Holmes/Rahe Social Readjustment Rating Scale

Life Event	Life Change Units
Death of a Spouse	100
Divorce	73
Marital Separation	65
Imprisonment	63
Death of a Close Family Member	63
Personal Injury or Illness	53
Marriage	50
Dismissal from Work	47
Marital Reconciliation	45
Retirement	45
Change in Health of Family Member	44
Pregnancy	40
Sexual Difficulties	39
Gain a New Family Member	39
Business Readjustment	39
Change in Financial State	38
Change in Frequency of Arguments.	35
Major Mortgage	32
Foreclosure of Mortgage or Loan	30
Change in Responsibilities at Work	29
Child Leaving Home	29
Trouble with In-Laws	29
Outstanding Personal Achievement	28
Spouse Starts or Stop Work	26
Begin or End School	26
Change in Living Conditions	25
Revision of Personal Habits	24
Trouble with Boss	23
Change in Working Hours or Conditions	20
Change in Residence	20
Change in Schools	20
Change in Recreation	19
Change in Church Activities	19
Change in Social Activities	18
Minor Mortgage or Loan	17
Change in Sleeping Habits	16
Change in Number of Family Reunions	15
Change in Eating Habits	15
Vacation	13
Christmas	12
Minor Violation of Law	11

The Apostle Paul withstood stresses most cannot imagine. J. B. Phillips translated Paul's stress list as follows: "In my travels I have been in constant danger from rivers and floods, from bandits, from my own countrymen, and from pagans. I have faced danger in city streets, danger in the desert, danger on the high seas, danger among false Christians. I have known exhaustion, pain, long vigils, hunger and thirst, doing without meals, cold and lack of clothing."[117] Paul should have been a nervous wreck, yet he never wavered.

He explained his unshakable faith and unflappable spirit in these words: "I am persuaded that neither death nor life, nor angels nor principalities nor powers, nor things present nor things to come, nor height nor depth, nor any other created thing, shall be able to separate us from the love of God which is in Christ Jesus our Lord."[118]

It is clear that Paul was constantly aware of God's presence. This is the sort of relationship described by Brother Lawrence, a humble kitchen worker, in *The Practice of the Presence of God*.[119] When one walks with God in the sunshine, His presence in the shadow is unmistakable.

A good deal of stress is self-inflicted. Worry and frustration extract a tremendous toll. For many years I have taught a simple, but effective, technique for reducing or eliminating the stress of worry and the feeling of being overwhelmed by the tasks at hand. I encourage anyone who is anxious or worried to purchase a small, pocket-sized notebook that can easily be carried at all times. Any time a concern arises or one discovers something that needs to be done, the concern or task is immediately written down in the notebook. This immediately removes the stress that results from trying to remember the item.

Once a day, at a convenient time, take out a blank sheet of paper. Draw a line down the center. On the left side write "can do" and on the right side "can't do" (Figure 1). Go through the notebook item by item, placing each in the appropriate column. Tasks such as "Wash clothes" or "Get the oil changed" are placed in the "can do" column because, given adequate time and resources,

Figure 1	Items of Concern
Can Do	**Can't Do**
Wash clothes	Make slow drivers move over
Get oil changed	Get troops out of Afghanistan
Complete job estimate	Stop terrorist attacks

you could personally wash the clothes and take the car in for servicing. Items such as "Slow drivers need to stay in the right lane" and "We need to get out of Afghanistan" are listed on the right side because no matter how much time you personally spend fussing or worrying about them the situation is unlikely to change.

Items in the "can do" list are then prioritized. This may be done simply by numbering them, but it is often more effective to take out a second sheet of paper and divide it into four quadrants by drawing lines down and across the page (Figure 2). Items are placed in the quadrants based upon two criteria: importance and urgency. Each item is then placed in the most appropriate quadrant, high importance–high urgency, high importance–low urgency, low importance–high urgency, and low importance–low urgency. In prioritizing, you will find that you become much more productive and satisfied if you concentrate on the items you have designated of high importance, even if they are of low urgency.

Figure 2	Priority List

High Importance–Urgent	**Low Importance–Urgent**
Complete job estimate	Answer the phone
High Importance–Non-urgent	**Low Importance–Non-urgent**
Get oil changed	Sweep the garage
Wash clothes	Organize the hall closet

This sort of priority matrix was used extensively by President Dwight D. Eisenhower, who is often quoted as saying, "What is important is seldom urgent and what is urgent is seldom important." It is believed that the concept was passed down to him by his mentor, Major General Fox Conner. The use of a priority matrix was later popularized by author Stephen Covey.

Much of the stress we experience is the result of responding to the countless number of "urgent" demands upon our time, regardless of their importance. It is very easy to become distracted by the ringing of the phone or a box full of e-mails and fail to accomplish a very important task because it does not carry the same sense of urgency. It is better to accomplish the important task and subsequently respond to messages than to accept all interruptions and leave the truly rewarding work undone.

A helpful phrase to remember is "Life is an Unfinishedness." If you are consistently writing things down as you think of them, you will never complete every item on your "can do" list. This is a perfectly normal situation. Having prepared for the day by organizing and prioritizing your tasks, however, you will experience the satisfaction that you have completed what was most necessary, given the time that was available.

After prioritizing the "can do" items, turn your attention to the "can't do" entries. Rather than continuing to invest time and energy into them, release them. This may be accomplished by crumpling the can't do list and tossing it into a waste basket or by consciously turning the items over to God, trusting that He will bring them to a suitable conclusion in His time.

Stress and the Adrenal Glands

How does stress affect longevity? While many factors are involved, the body's stress response depends greatly upon two small triangular glands called the adrenals. The term adrenal derives from the glands' location (*Ad* means "next to" and *renal* refers to the kidney). The glands sit atop the kidneys.

Adrenal glands are comprised of two parts. The inner portion, called the medulla, is responsible for producing and releasing the chemicals that control the body's response to threats, the "fight and flight response." These hormones are called adrenaline (epinephrine) and noradrenaline (norepinephrine).

The actions of adrenaline and noradrenaline are often identical. Both increase the heart rate and open air passages. Both cause blood vessels in non-essential areas to narrow, causing a rise in blood pressure. Both cause the pupils to dilate.

Adrenaline elevates blood sugar by increasing the formation of glucose in the liver. It also causes fats to begin to break down for energy production. It inhibits non-essential activities such as digestion and the immune system's response to challenges. Noradrenaline plays an important role in the transmission of nerve impulses. This is important in preventing anxiety and depression.

The outer portion of the gland, called the cortex, manufactures at least twenty-five hormones, of three different classes. Mineralcorticoids such as aldosterone regulate the body's fluid and electrolyte balance. Androgens including dihydroepiandosterone (DHEA), testosterone, progesterone, and estrogen augment the hormonal production of the testes or ovaries.

The adrenal cortex also produces glucocorticoids, of which cortisol (cortisone) is the best known. Cortisol helps maintain blood pressure and regulates the breakdown of proteins, fats, and carbohydrates. It also blocks the immune system's inflammatory response to injury. Cortisol acts to maintain the body's response to stress.

When exposed to a stressful event, such as meeting an unrestrained Doberman Pincer in the middle of a morning walk, the adrenal medulla springs into action and secretes adrenaline and noradrenaline. If the threat lasts more than a few minutes, the adrenal cortex is called in to assist and cortisol levels rise.

The stress response is designed to be of short duration. It is designed with the expectation that one of two things will happen quickly. Either the threat will be successfully eliminated or death will occur. A prolonged shutdown of "noncritical" bodily functions is neither expected nor intended.

Unfortunately, many people find themselves under constant, unmanaged stress. If this stress is not addressed regularly by the methods presented earlier in this chapter, it will become chronic and adversely affect adrenal activity. You will reach a point at which adrenaline and noradrenaline are no longer required simply to fight or run, but to keep going. Cortisol will remain elevated to keep on top of the perceived threat.

Doctors recognize two diseases caused by adrenal dysfunction. One is Cushing's syndrome, which is caused by sustained levels of abnormally high cortisol. This is usually due to a hormone-secreting tumor. Cushing's syndrome is characterized by upper body weight gain, thinning of the skin, easy bruising, loss of bone strength, fatigue, muscle weakness, hypertension, diabetes, loss of sex drive, increased irritability, anxiety, and depression.

The other disease recognized by physicians is adrenal failure, which is called Addison's disease. Addison's disease is characterized by chronic fatigue, muscle weakness, weight loss, low blood pressure, a darkening of the skin, increased irritability, depression, craving for salty foods due to increased salt loss, irregular menses, and hypoglycemic (low blood sugar) episodes.

There is, however, a third condition that is not currently an acceptable medical diagnosis. It is, therefore, rarely addressed. That entity is adrenal fatigue.

Adrenal fatigue is not defined by the abnormally high cortisol levels of Cushing's syndrome, nor is it characterized by the extremely low hormonal levels of Addison's disease. Adrenal fatigue is a condition in which the adrenal glands have become unable to keep up with the demands placed upon them. This places the body at risk of disease development or premature aging.

Many symptoms are suggestive of adrenal fatigue. The most common are extreme exhaustion, failing to awake refreshed after a full night's sleep, and the presence of what is often referred to as a "brain fog." Because adrenal fatigue often goes unrecognized, I developed the Adrenal Fatigue Quiz at the end of this chapter. If you are having difficulty getting through the day the quiz will tell you whether adrenal fatigue should be considered.

Adrenal fatigue may occur when the body has required adrenal hormones to sustain the stress response for a prolonged period of time. It may be caused by a deficiency in the nutrients required for hormone production. In most cases it is a combination of both; the adrenals are often overworked and underpaid.

It follows, therefore, that if normal adrenal function is to be restored, the demands placed upon the glands must be lessened and the resources available to them must be increased. Doing one without the other is unlikely to resolve the challenge.

Stress Reduction

Stress must be reduced at home and in the workplace. This involves four distinct steps. The first step is to improve the quality of rest being received. This will be addressed in chapter fifteen.

Secondly, interpersonal conflicts must be resolved. This often involves improving communication. One of the leading causes of strained relationships is the misattribution of a motive by one of the parties.

For example, one individual related that he became resentful of his supervisor when he heard her mutter "That figures!" after he had reported that a project had been delayed. He assumed that the comment had been directed at him—that she had made the comment because she believed him to be slow and incompetent. As time passed, he found his job infinitely more stressful and reporting to work each day increasingly difficult.

Finally, he decided to confront his supervisor about the remark. He learned that his supervisor actually valued his work highly and believed him to be an excellent employee. The remark had nothing to do with his job performance. It was simply that when he reported the delay she was near the end of a day in which nothing had gone as expected. Since the delay matched the rest of her day, she had reacted by saying "That figures." She apologized for making the remark without thinking about his reaction and he for jumping to the wrong conclusion. Their relationship was restored and he experienced renewed enthusiasm for his work.

The third step in easing stress is to clear non-essential events from the schedule. When you have too much on your plate the best solution is to remove some of the items. This may mean asking to be released from some commitments. It may mean not traveling to a nephew's wedding or not participating in a community service project. While stepping back is difficult, it is essential to recovery.

The fourth step is closely related to the third. You must learn to say "no." It is of no value to remove one event from your schedule only to fill it with another. This may even apply to a project at work. Although uncomfortable, it is much better to explain to an employer that you are not up to the task than to explain why you failed to complete it or did a poor job.

It is extremely important to discontinue the use of chemical stimulants, even if symptoms increase when doing so. Caffeinated coffees, teas, and soft drinks should be replaced by pure water or other non-caffeinated beverages. Stimulatory herbs such as guarana, bitter orange, and panax ginseng should be avoided. Pep pills, including those that contain decongestants like pseudoephedrine, should also be avoided.

An additional step to reduce mental or emotional stress is to break the news habit. Newspapers, newsmagazines, broadcast news programs, and radio and television talk shows are incredibly rich sources of "can't do" items that do little but drain our emotional energy. It is far more helpful to read and listen to encouraging and uplifting books, tapes, and CDs, which build rather than drain one's emotional bank account.

Supporting the Body's Stress Response

Support of the body is also important. As with the spirit and the mind, this should be an ongoing process, not something that is begun when the stressful event appears.

Regular physical activity, which keeps the body conditioned, enables the body to respond to stress efficiently. Getting the body moving and keeping it moving for twenty to thirty minutes three to five times weekly is ideal for most people. Those with conditions such as diabetes are encouraged to do so on a daily basis.

A comprehensive supplement that provides optimum levels of all vitamins, minerals, and essential amino acids should be taken daily. Essential fatty acids, which are critical for proper brain function, should also be provided. These are commonly found in vegetable oils such as flax oil, borage oil, or evening primrose oil and in oils derived from the belly fat of cold-water fishes. These are not fish liver oils, but those commonly referred to as Omega-3s.

In times of stress, the body's demand for B vitamins increases. This may explain why many people develop a craving for carbohydrates during times of stress. B vitamins are found in complex carbohydrates such as whole grains, but are stripped away during the refining process. Ironically, increasing one's intake of refined carbohydrates further increases the demand for B vitamins and decreases the body's ability to cope with the challenge that is present.

Vitamin B-5, pantothenic acid, is particularly critical during times of stress because the body needs it to produce a critical substance called Coenzyme A. Coenzyme A is required for energy production and is also essential in the manufacture of stress hormones such as cortisol and adrenaline. Low levels of Coenzyme A will severely limit the body's ability to withstand stress and can lead to extreme tiredness and fatigue.

Because B vitamins are water-soluble, they cannot be stored in the body. They must be administered at least twice daily. Another water-soluble nutrient is vitamin C. The demand for vitamin C increases dramatically during times of stress and it, like the B vitamins, must be taken at least twice daily for optimum benefit.

A number of herbal substances are capable of enhancing the body's ability to respond to stress by modulating the activity of the nervous system. Many have been demonstrated to calm anxiety and enhance relaxation while actually increasing the ability to concentrate and react appropriately to stimuli.

Some of the herbs commonly used in stress management include valerian, skullcap, chamomile, and hops. I prefer combinations rather than single herb preparations. In my experience, herbal combinations, which typically contain lower amounts of each ingredient than when they are used as single agents, work more smoothly and effectively and have a very low incidence of side effects.

Stress is unavoidable. It is as much a part of life as eating, breathing, or sleeping. You will always experience challenges. Stress need not be feared, however. If you are diligent in supporting your physical, emotional, and spiritual needs you will be up to the challenge, whenever or however it comes.

When you are adequately prepared, you will welcome stress, for you will find yourself energized and driven to new levels of achievement by its presence. Once you are able to embrace stress as a friend, you will find that it is really nothing but an additional source of energy. You will be able to say with Helen Keller, "Life is either a grand adventure or it is nothing."[120]

Adrenal Fatigue Quiz

- Do you feel excessively fatigued?
- Would you describe yourself as physically and emotionally exhausted?
- Do you feel just as bad as or worse than the night before when you awaken after a full night's sleep?
- Do you feel overwhelmed or unable to cope?
- Do you crave salty foods?
- Are you irritable or do you cry easily?
- Would you have trouble functioning without coffee, cola, or a "pep pill"?
- Do you feel more energetic in the evening than earlier in the day?
- Is your stamina low?
- Does exercise leave you feeling drained for hours or days?
- Do you seem to "catch" every cold or flu bug that comes your way?
- Are injuries slow to heal?
- Do illnesses seem to drag on indefinitely?
- Do you have difficulty concentrating as though you are living in a "brain fog"?
- Have you lost you sex drive?
- Do you suffer from poor digestion?
- Are you having more allergy symptoms than usual?
- Do you struggle more with premenstrual syndrome than you did in the past or, if menopausal, are you having more hot flashes or other symptoms?
- Has your blood pressure been low?
- Are you extremely sensitive to cold?

Scoring:

5 or less "yes" answers: Adrenal fatigue is unlikely

6 – 10 "yes" answers: Adrenal fatigue may be present

11 – 15 "yes" answers: You probably have significant adrenal fatigue

16 – 20 "yes" answers: You almost certainly are experiencing severe adrenal fatigue

Chapter 13

Renew Your Mind

And do not be conformed to this world, but be transformed by the renewing of your mind, that you may prove what is that good and acceptable and perfect will of God.
– Romans 12:2

Defining the Mind

It is impossible to overestimate the incredible faculties of the human mind. When I speak of the mind, I am not referring to the brain. The brain is a physical organ; it is capable of being injured or becoming diseased. The brain stores memories and coordinates an infinite number of processes within the body, but it is not synonymous with the mind.

The mind is different than the brain. Unlike the brain, the mind survives the death of the body as evidenced by the ability of survivors of near death experiences to recount the details of activities being conducted during their resuscitation. The mind governs our activities to the point of determining our time of death.

Evidence of this is seen in the increase of death rates following holidays and other important events. For example, Thomas Jefferson, John Adams, and James Monroe all died on July 4th. Clearly, they willed themselves to live until the anniversary of the event that was central to their lives and then gave up the fight. Deaths in New York City were up 50 percent during the first week of 2000 as individuals who had determined to see the turn of the century released their hold on life.[121]

I have personally known people who willed themselves to live or die. I once hospitalized an elderly woman for treatment of pneumonia. Her condition was not serious, and I anticipated that she would fully recover. As the days passed it appeared that all was progressing well. Her fever broke and her breathing became easier. Her chest x-ray showed that the infection was resolving. On a Wednesday morning, I advised her to expect to be discharged on the following day. Completely unexpectedly, and without any discernable cause, she died that night.

A week later her daughter-in-law came to my office. "I have to ask you a question," she began. "Was there a reason that my mother-in-law died last Wednesday?"

"None that I've been able to determine," I replied, explaining that her mother-in-law's condition had improved to the point that I had planned to discharge her Thursday morning.

"I thought so," the woman continued. "As I was getting ready to leave her room that evening she asked me, 'Did Dr. Peterson say that I have pneumonia?' to which I replied, 'Yes, he did.' My mother-in-law then said quietly, 'Hmmm, that could be my ticket out of here.' She died a few hours later."

On the other extreme, I once participated in the care of a young woman who had developed breast cancer. The cancer had spread throughout her body, including to her brain and to her bones. One morning her left hip, in which the bone had been replaced by tumor, broke as she rolled over in bed. It could not be repaired because there was no bone to work with. With the cancer being so widespread, I believed that death was imminent. I did not tell her so, but I did not expect her to survive longer than one or two more weeks. Incredibly, she lived another two years solely on her desire to be present for her children.

The Conscious and the Subconscious Mind

The mind has two levels, the conscious and the subconscious. The conscious mind is our level of awareness; it is the center of our thought and reason. The subconscious mind functions behind the scenes. It contains programs, some of which are basic to our survival and others that have arisen from our life experience. The subconscious mind is programmed primarily by the input of others during our childhood. If the dominant messages received are positive, such as "You are so smart; I know you'll do great in school," the child will be programmed to perform well in school. If, on the other hand, the dominant messages are "You're stupid—you'll never amount to anything!" the child will likely become a dropout and struggle with life.

Subconscious programs run on autopilot. Sadly, most people are completely unaware of their presence. Ignorance, however, is often not bliss. I have known women, for example, that go from one abusive relationship to another because they have a subconscious program running that says they are not worthy of true love and affection. They may consciously desire a kind, gentle, loving husband, but when a subconscious program is in conflict with a conscious desire, the subconscious always wins.

The good news is that subconscious programs can be changed, allowing one's life to take a new direction. The elements of change are recognition, repetition, and emotion. It is critically important to renew your subconscious mind because subconscious programs can lead to disease and even death. I know from personal experience.

The Power of Subconscious Programming

In the fall of 2001, a profound change occurred in my life. I couldn't put my finger on what was wrong, but it was clear that something was amiss. Although I was consciously smiling, I was frequently told, "You should smile more often." I would make recommendations to people consulting with me, but they wouldn't follow through. It was as though they hadn't really heard what I had said.

In seeking an answer, I found myself attending a series of workshops conducted by Brian Klemmer and Associates.[122] Brian is an expert in recognizing and dealing with subconscious programming. During one of the sessions, we attendees were asked to define a mission statement for the workshop. As the debate wore on, I stood and gave what I considered to be a helpful insight into the process. Amazingly, discussion continued where it had left off before I stood to speak. It was as though no one was aware of my presence in the room.

Later that day, we were asked to do an exercise in which we recalled our interaction with our parents. During the exercise I suddenly recognized what had happened to me. When my father died of a heart attack at age fifty-four I had no idea how to prevent the same outcome in my own life. A subconscious program began running that said I would die of a heart attack by the time I was fifty-four years old. In October 2001 I turned fifty-four. I had not died of a heart attack because in the intervening years I had discovered the mechanism that causes plaque to build up in arteries and had taken steps to stop the process. The subconscious program had continued to run, however. When I turned fifty-four it activated and I died emotionally. I was still physically alive, but my emotional energy was so low that others could not really "see" me.

That evening the point was driven home in a most dramatic fashion. We workshop attendees were asked to participate in an exercise called "The Samurai Game." The setting was medieval Japan and opposing samurai armies were facing each other. Combat would be conducted by exercises such as "Rock, Paper, Scissors" and tests of balance. One of the ground rules was that the team leaders could not look any of the facilitators directly in the eye. Before the action started my team leader looked the lead facilitator in the eye and was told that he must kill one of his warriors. Without hesitation he turned, pointed directly at me and said, "Dale, you're dead."

I was told to go lie in the "cemetery" with my eyes closed while the game commenced. What a vivid metaphor for what I had been experiencing over the previous six months. I was "dead," but aware of the many activities of life going on all around me.

Having recognized the existence of the subconscious program and experienced strong emotions regarding its existence, I was immediately able to replace it with a program that supported my desire to live a full and rewarding life.

In my workshops, I have people perform activities that demonstrate the incredible power of the mind. They see firsthand how their mind can overcome seemingly insurmountable obstacles, how it can take them beyond their perceived limits.

Effectively managing subconscious programs is a key element in the quest to achieve and maintain optimum wellness. Doing so is an ongoing challenge, but you are instructed to do so. You are not to be conformed to this world, going blindly through life making decisions based upon subconscious programs put in place by parents, teachers, and others in your formative years. You are to be transformed by the renewing of your mind. You are challenged to live up to your full potential.

Chapter 14

Become a Spiritual Warrior

For we do not wrestle against flesh and blood, but against principalities, against
powers, against the rulers of the darkness of this age,
against spiritual hosts of wickedness in the heavenly places.
– Ephesians 6:12

When a subject exists that people are loath to discuss, it is often referred to as "the elephant in the room." It is something that is too big to go unnoticed, but it is also something that no one is willing to admit seeing. There is an elephant in the sick room; it is the existence of spiritual entities that are capable of adversely affecting the health of human beings.

The Reality of Spiritual Entities

The existence of such entities has been recognized by nearly all societies since the dawn of time. Witch doctors, medicine men, and shamans practice their healing arts primarily in the spiritual realm. One of the most revealing pictures of the spirit world is given by Jungleman of the Yanomamö tribe that lives in Venezuela's rain forest. He relates his experiences and those of another shaman, Chief Shoefoot, in *Spirit of the Rainforest: A Yanomamo Shaman's Story.*[123]

Raised to be a shaman from childhood, Chief Shoefoot became adept at seeing and responding to spiritual entities. Through the use of drugs and chants he was able to call spirits to help him become a great healer. Over time, however, he realized that the spirits were killing people rather than healing them. He also recognized that they were trying to destroy him as well. He was aware of Yai Pada, the Great Spirit, who dwells in a place of light surrounded by other beings who are praising Him, but he was afraid to chant to Him because the other spirits had told him that Yai Pada was his enemy. Finally, in an act of desperation, he called out to the Great Spirit to help him. He testifies that the evil spirits who were holding him captive fled and have never returned.

Chief Shoefoot's experience with evil spirits is not unique. While I was in medical school, I attended luncheons sponsored by the Christian Medical Society. The talks were frequently given by physicians who were serving or had served as medical missionaries in foreign countries. We students would listen with interest to their stories of dealing with diseases brought on by the activity of evil spirits, and we would ask why, if such entities existed, we did not see them in the United States.

In the fall of 1997, Chief Shoefoot came to the United States on a speaking tour. While here, he stated that he sensed greater spiritual danger on American streets than in his native jungle. "I can see evil spirits' footprints all over this place," he told his host, "but you don't see them."[124]

There are two possible explanations as to why we medical students did not see evidence of evil spirits influencing disease in 1970 and why Chief Shoefoot saw them all over the United States in 1997. The first is that we were blind to their presence; they were at work, but we were not able to see them. The second is that the activity of evil spirits in the United States was not as great thirty years prior to Chief Shoefoot's visit. I believe that the latter is true.

I did not encounter what I considered activity of evil spirits in disease until I had been in practice for many years. In retrospect, I believe it was because in 1970 the United States was still a predominantly Christian nation. As the country turned from Christianity to paganism over the succeeding decades, evidence of the influence of spiritual entities on the health of individuals increased dramatically. I now encounter such activity with regularity.

Spiritual Entities and Health Challenges

At times, the role of a spiritual entity is obvious. This is when an individual is manifesting dramatic physical symptoms despite completely normal physical findings. I was once consulted by a woman who was suffering from intense shortness of breath. She had seen many physicians and had undergone extensive testing, but the cause of her breathing difficulty could not be found.

As we talked, I learned that just prior to the onset of her shortness of breath she had taken on the job of demolishing an abandoned shack. She had not experienced any trauma or difficulty during the project and she had gone to bed that evening feeling fine. She awoke, however, with intense shortness of breath that had never eased or gone away. She confided that since that time she had heard audible voices while driving her truck.

I asked her if she believed in God. She answered that she had asked Jesus to be her personal savior at an early age, but that she had not taken that relationship seriously for quite some time. I asked her if she was willing to confirm her relationship with Jesus Christ and she did so. I then asked her if she was willing to command any spirit that was causing her shortness of breath to leave. She was willing and did so. She awoke the following morning able to breathe freely for the first time since the shortness of breath had appeared.

Most of the time, however, the influence of spiritual entities is not so obvious. That is because they are not causing the health challenge; they are simply amplifying its intensity. This is a phenomenon reported by Chief Shoefoot. He discovered that when sick people came seeking his help, the spirits he was relying upon would often cause the illness to become more severe. When the effect of a condition on a person's life appears to be greater than what would be predicted or when a medical condition does not respond to treatment as it should, it is quite likely that a spiritual entity is involved and needs to be addressed.

Societies have different names for spirit entities. In the Ojibwe language they are called *totems*. In Chinese the word is *tuteng*, in Korean it is *jangseung*, and the Polish term is *rodnidze*. Hindus speak of *grahas*, and the Irish of *banshees*. Many in modern Western societies refer to them as "spirit guides." The English Bible refers to them as demons, from the Greek word *daimones*.

During Jesus' earthly ministry He taught, healed the sick, and cast out demons. It is important to note that sickness did not automatically mean demonic activity. There were many instances in which a physical or mental ailment was cured without any action being taken in regard to a spirit, and there were cases in which a demon was ordered to leave someone who was not exhibiting any signs of illness.

The Bible depicts evil spirits as members of a spiritual army. The commander-in-chief is referred to as Satan, the devil, or Beelzebub. There are several ranks including principalities (*arches*), powers (*exousias*), and rulers of darkness (*kosmokratoras tou skotous*). This army is characterized by spiritual wickedness.

It is difficult for someone who has a relationship with a seemingly benign "spirit guide" or "guardian angel" to believe that the entity would ever do them harm. Nevertheless, just as the spirit guides who came to Chief Shoefoot as beautiful creatures subsequently sought to destroy him, so friendly and attractive spirit guides may ultimately seek to destroy the health and even take the life of their human host. I recall a beautiful young girl who attempted to take her own life and that of her parents because a spirit who called himself Jesus was audibly telling her to do so.

Dealing with Spiritual Entities

Many techniques have been developed for dealing with evil spirits. Garlic has been used to ward off evil spirits for millennia. Ancient Egyptians hung wreaths of garlic in children's rooms to protect them from having their breath taken by evil spirits. Greek midwives hung bags of garlic in delivery rooms to prevent spirits from attacking the babies. Cultures as diverse as China, Malaysia, and the West Indies still use garlic to protect against evil spirits.

Elaborate rituals have been devised for freeing a person from the hold of an evil spirit. The Roman Catholic Church, for example, has a rite of exorcism, which is conducted by a priest. The ritual is detailed in an 84-page Latin document, "De Exorcismus et Supplicationibus Quibusdam" ("Of All Kinds of Exorcisms and Supplications"). A Roman Catholic exorcism was the focal point of the 1973 movie *The Exorcist*. Many Protestant denominations have much attenuated instructions for exorcisms. A wide array of "deliverance ministries" have sprung up which, while they do not necessarily follow a set ritual, often put on theatrical performances in which conversations are carried on with the spirit or spirits, a cross or Bible is used as a prop, and much shouting takes place.

Rituals and theatrical performances are not necessary to deal with spiritual entities. I know energy workers who have success in eliminating the effects of spiritual entities very quietly and with no drama whatsoever. Nowhere in the Bible is there an instance in which an elaborate ritual was used to deal with a spiritual entity. Neither is there any account of a shouting match between Jesus or His apostles and a demon. I have taught many parents that if they find themselves in a shouting match with one of their children they have lost control of the situation. The same is true of a self-proclaimed exorcist that finds himself in a shouting match with a spirit.

When a spiritual entity is adversely affecting the health of an individual, only two things are required. First and foremost, the afflicted individual must want to be freed from the effects being exerted by the spirit. In situations in which the person is obtaining benefit from the entity's presence (receiving guidance or insight) or in which the person is living in fear of the spirit, there may be a reluctance to express a desire that the offending spirit leave. In those instances, effort should be placed on bringing the individual to the point of seeing the need to be free of the spirit's influence rather than on commanding the entity to leave. It is extremely difficult, perhaps impossible, to free someone from the effects of a malevolent spirit if that person does not want to sever the relationship.

Once an individual has expressed a desire to be free of the influence of a spiritual entity, all that is required is for the individual to command the spirit to leave using the authority given them by Jesus Christ. There is no specific formula. Chief Shoefoot simply cried out to *Yai Pada*, the Great Spirit, to help him escape the bonds of the spirits within him. The one true God exerts authority over the spiritual realm and evil spirits must obey Him. The spirits of the Yanomamö refer to Him as *Yai Wana Naba Laywa*, the "unfriendly enemy spirit."

What is commonly referred to as demon possession, in which a spirit or spirits have been invited to enter a human body and allowed to exert their control, is not nearly as common as external attacks from those entities. Many Christians have a naïve view of the spirit world. They profess belief in a Holy Spirit and even in angels, but they often deny the existence of unholy spirits. Most who do accept the reality of evil or unholy spirits mistakenly believe that once they have accepted Jesus Christ as their personal Savior they are immune to the activities of those spirit beings.

Nothing could be further from the truth! The more committed one becomes to serving Jesus Christ, the more likely he or she is to experience an attack by an evil or unholy spirit. The Bible explicitly states that a war is going on in another dimension. After the prophet Daniel had been in mourning for a period of three weeks, he saw an angelic being. The angel told Daniel that he had started to come to him at the outset, but had been stopped by an opposing spiritual being, the "prince of Persia" (Daniel was living in Persia at the time).[125] The spirit had needed to call upon his general, Michael, to help him break through the enemy lines and reach Daniel.

In Ephesians 6:12, the Apostle Paul informs his readers that they are engaged in a spiritual battle, that they are participants in a war that is taking place in the spiritual dimension. He tells them that the challenges they are encountering in the material world are actually originating in a spiritual dimension. "We wrestle not," he writes, "against flesh and blood," but against a spiritual army. Wrestling implies a personal, intimate, one-on-one contest. While many Christians today believe they can hire professional clergy to do their fighting for them, the Bible makes clear the fact that every true follower of Jesus Christ must engage in spiritual warfare.

A Christian who takes his or her faith seriously will be attacked by unholy spirits. This is logical, for a soldier on the front lines in a war zone is far more likely to come under enemy fire than someone like me who is living comfortably in the interior of the United States. When such attacks come, as they inevitably will, it is important to face them. "Resist the devil," we are told in James 4:7, "and he will flee from you."

How can a follower of Jesus Christ resist a member of Satan's army? (I say a member of his army because the devil is not omnipresent. He creates the battle plan, but he has greater things to do than personally attack individuals. The Commander in Chief of the Armed Forces does not enter into hand to hand combat with an enemy soldier.) A Christian resists a spiritual being by telling it to leave by the authority he or she has in Christ. When Jesus was confronted with a demon, He did not pull out the Star of David. He simply told the entity to leave. When He sent out seventy of His followers in advance of His coming to various towns and cities, they returned with joy saying, "Lord, even the demons are subject to us in Your name."[126]

That is an important statement. It contains a truth that is missed by many. The demons were subject to *them*, Christ's disciples. Yes, the devil and his demons are subject to God and they are subject to Jesus Christ, but they are also subject to His representatives on earth—to those who claim the name of Jesus.

Lest someone argue that this authority over spiritual entities was limited to Jesus' closest disciples, Jesus' words as He taught His disciples how He would go away and come again need to be considered. He said, "For the Son of man is as a man taking a far journey, who left his house, and gave authority to his servants, and to every man his work, and commanded the porter to watch."[127] Jesus likened His ascension to Heaven to a man going on a long journey and leaving his servants in charge of the household. The man gave them authority to act in his absence. So Jesus has given His servants on earth the authority to act in His physical absence.

It has been my experience that while all evil spirits are subject to the authority of Jesus' servants on earth, some are more likely to challenge that authority than are others. The most tenacious are those that have been invited into a person either intentionally, as in the case of Chief Shoefoot, or tacitly through actions such as using mind-altering drugs or dabbling in the occult. Since they believe that they have a right to be present, they will resist the command to leave until the person with whom they are associated makes it clear that they are no longer welcome.

Only slightly less obstinate are spirits who have participated in theatrical displays or shouting matches characteristic of many deliverance ministries. They know that someone who feels the need to use a wooden cross or shout is not confident in his or her authority to demand that a spirit leave. I have seen individuals who have sought deliverance on several occasions only to find that the oppressive spirit was still present. Exorcism rituals, it seems, are an interesting game to be played between humans and demons, but they lack the effectiveness of the exercise of true authority.

It is essential that servants of Jesus Christ understand the authority vested in them. The phrase "in Jesus' name" is not a magic incantation like "abracadabra" or "open sesame." It is an affirmation of the basis upon which one's authority rests. It is akin to a police officer telling a suspect to "stop in the name of the law." He is telling the suspected criminal that his authority to demand that he stop is rooted in the law, and therefore has substance. A police officer possesses the full authority of the law to make an arrest; a servant of Jesus Christ holds the full authority to order an evil spirit to leave.

In nearly all instances in which that authority is exercised with confidence and assurance, a spirit that has been adversely affecting a person's health will leave immediately. Some spirits, however, will resist that authority, just as some criminals will resist arrest. On one occasion some of Jesus' disciples encountered a demon that refused to leave. They asked Jesus why they had been unsuccessful in commanding it to stop afflicting a child. He responded, "This kind can come out by nothing but prayer and fasting."[128]

I remember vividly an occasion in which a spirit refused to stop afflicting a young girl who had been taken to a deliverance ministry prior to consulting with me. I did not lack confidence, but despite the fact that the spirit had been told to leave, the girl's severe symptoms continued unabated. Her condition required hospitalization and standard medical treatment for stabilization. I asked many others to pray while I continued to wrestle with what I knew was an evil spirit causing the girl's condition. After three days, I felt a release in my spirit. Despite having what is considered an incurable condition, she quickly improved. She was off all "lifelong" medications within two months, she successfully returned to college, and she has been free of all signs and symptoms of the disease since that time (a period of over four years to date).

One may reasonably ask how it can be determined that a spirit being is adversely affecting a person's health. There are two extremes of thought in this regard. There are some who attribute all illness to the presence of spiritual forces in people's lives. On the other side are those who do not believe that spiritual entities exist, who consider the Biblical account of demonic activity and the work of shamans and witch doctors to be rooted in fantasy and superstition.

A careful reading of Scripture, an open analysis of history, and present day experience all lead to the conclusion that the truth is between the two extreme views. Evil spirits are not the root cause of all disease. They do, however, exist and are capable of causing or intensifying physical illness in human beings. Determining whether a spiritual entity is actively affecting a disease process is not a matter of guesswork. When one becomes sensitive to the existence of beings in the spiritual dimension, their presence can be recognized. Suspicion that a spiritual entity is at work can be confirmed while running a computer system check as discussed in Chapter 11.

Spirit beings do exist, and they are active in human affairs. It is naïve to think otherwise. They need not be viewed with awe or feared because as believers in God and servants of Jesus Christ they are subject to our authority. Spiritual attacks are not the usual cause of physical or mental illness, but the possibility must be entertained and addressed appropriately if optimum health is to be achieved.

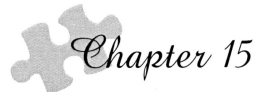

Chapter 15

Factors You Control That Determine Your Level of Wellness

Therefore we do not lose heart. Even though our outward man is perishing,
yet the inward man is being renewed day by day.
– 2 Corinthians 4:16

Far too many people, physicians included, approach life believing that disease "just happens," that whether one becomes sick or dies prematurely is simply a matter of chance. "I have bad genes," someone might say. "I've sure been unlucky when it comes to my health," another might muse.

Genetic factors, which are uncontrollable and cannot be changed, do cause some diseases to predictably appear. Cystic fibrosis, Down's syndrome, and Huntington's chorea are examples of conditions that are genetically predetermined. Most genetic codes, however, simply predispose to disease development; they do not dictate that a disease will appear. Type 2 diabetes mellitus, coronary artery disease, cancer, and connective tissue disorders are examples of diseases for which an individual may be genetically predisposed, but which are determined to a much greater degree by environmental factors and personal choices.

Controllable factors play a far greater role in determining a person's level of wellness than pre-set genetic factors. Those controllable factors have been detailed in previous chapters, but it is well to review them to give an overview of what can be done to enhance the chance of living a long and productive life.

The Quality of Air You Breathe

The first factor is the quality of air you breathe. Do not underestimate the adverse effects of cigarette smoking on the body. I once saw a man in his early seventies who presented with signs and symptoms of end-stage emphysema. He reported that he had begun smoking cigarettes as a child and had averaged between two and three packs daily over the course of his life. Total exposure to cigarette smoke is measured in pack-years. Smoking one pack of cigarettes daily for one year is equivalent to one pack-year. While the average individual begins to show evidence of smoking related disease after twenty to thirty pack-years, this man had managed to tolerate in excess of 160 pack-years! He could have been the poster-boy for why cigarette smoking is harmless. The rest of the story, however, is that he was about to become the first person on either side of his family to die prior to the age of ninety. His decision to smoke cigarettes had shortened his life by nearly twenty years!

What You Put into Your Body

Consider what you put into your body. Health can be destroyed quickly through the use of drugs, but it can also be destroyed slowly by consuming small amounts of toxic food additives and preservatives each day.

New amalgam fillings should be avoided. What are commonly referred to as silver fillings aren't really silver. They are made up of a combination of approximately 50 percent mercury combined with smaller amounts of silver, copper, tin, and sometimes other metals like zinc. Mercury is a toxic substance that has been removed from most products in the marketplace. Some dentists and governmental agencies continue to insist that mercury amalgams are perfectly safe, but I find it difficult to accept their conclusion when other governmental agencies continually warn against mercury exposure.

Pure water is essential to good health, but carbonated beverages cause a loss of bone strength by requiring the body to neutralize the acid they contain. Diets high in refined foods can promote the development of diabetes, while eating a diet rich in fruits, vegetables, and other whole foods promotes long-term health.

Giving your body quality nutritional supplementation is essential. Quality manufacturers analyze raw materials as they arrive at the plant, use only the most bioavailable forms of nutrients, follow pharmaceutical-grade manufacturing practices, and assay each lot for quality and purity before releasing it for sale.

What You Put onto Your Body

What you put onto your body is another factor you control in determining your state of health. The skin is highly absorbent. Drugs, particularly hormones, are often prescribed to be used topically, reaching the bloodstream through the skin. Toxic chemicals are also absorbed when they come in contact with the skin. Examples include solvents, cleaning supplies, chlorine from water, perfumes, cosmetics, and aluminum-containing antiperspirants.

The skin requires protection. Wear appropriate clothing and use sunscreen when spending long periods of time in the summer sun. The skin also requires nutrients, including emollients that soften the skin and vitamins, especially antioxidants, that help skin cells deal with the challenges they face from the environment.

Your health is determined to a great extent by the electromagnetic fields you encounter. You are constantly exposed to radio waves, television waves, microwaves, and waves from electronic appliances. Do not neglect the use of electromagnetic protection, which provides a measure of control over EMF exposure.

The Activities You Pursue

The activities you pursue also play a role in determining your state of health. Pursuing dangerous activities such as diving into water of unknown depth, not wearing recommended protective gear, driving too fast for road conditions, playing "Russian Roulette," or taking mind-altering drugs can irreversibly damage health in an instant. Other activities can damage health over time.

Taking prescription or over-the-counter drugs can seriously impair one's health. The Physician's Desk Reference, commonly referred to as the PDR, is a large volume measuring 10.9 x 8.8 x 3.2 inches and containing 3,500 pages. The font size is smaller than that found in most books. A large percentage of the PDR contents are the listings of the complications and adverse effects known to potentially arise from use of the drugs detailed in the book. Since physicians commonly fail to recognize symptoms reported to them by patients as due to drug side effects, it is imperative that anyone taking a drug become educated about the potential consequences of doing so. Websites such as www.drugs.com, www.rxlist.com, and www.drugwatch.com offer listings of common side effects for most medications.

Although rarely considered a potential health risk, television viewing can adversely affect one's health. Education and income level is inversely related to the number of hours spent watching television daily. Compared to one hour per day viewers, four hour per day viewers are more obese, more likely to smoke cigarettes, carry more hostility, and perform less physical activity.[129] Television viewing has been associated with depression, alcohol abuse, attention deficit hyperactivity disorder (ADHD), childhood leukemia, epilepsy, and diabetes.

Potentially harmful activities also include those for which you are not adequately prepared. The "Weekend Warrior" or occasional athlete is much more likely to be injured or have a heart attack than someone who exercises regularly and is in condition to participate in competitive athletic activities. It is important to avoid activities that your body cannot withstand. If you have osteopenia or osteoporosis (bone weakness), you should not take roller coaster rides or walk across uneven terrain where you are at risk of falling.

Just as you should avoid potentially harmful activities, there are beneficial activities that you should pursue. Flossing and brushing your teeth regularly can enable you to keep your teeth throughout your lifetime; loss of teeth can lead to difficulty eating nutritious foods such as fresh fruits, so protecting your teeth is important to your long-term health. The importance of getting your body moving for thirty minutes three to five times weekly has been discussed. Reading good books is associated with a higher education and income as well as better overall health and longevity.

The Quality of Rest You Receive

The next factor you control is the quality of rest you receive. There are many aspects to obtaining adequate rest. Ask any child to name his or her favorite time of the school day and you are likely to get the response "Recess!" Adults can also benefit from breaks during the workday.

Following a relaxing routine for thirty to sixty minutes prior to going to bed can result in getting to sleep more quickly and experiencing a more refreshing sleep. Few people today get an adequate amount of sleep. While today many people feel that six or seven hours of sleep is more than adequate, prior to the advent of electricity the average individual got 9 hours of sleep each night. There is an easy way to determine whether or not you are getting enough sleep. If you are getting an adequate amount of sleep you will not need an alarm to wake up.

One- to three-day retreats or "Get Aways" are another important element of rest. An example is seen in the Bible. Every time Jesus dealt with large groups of people or performed a major work, He retreated to the Mount of Olives or to the opposite side of the Sea of Galilee. Taking a short retreat every six to twelve weeks seems to be a good routine. Finally, a significant break from work responsibilities should be taken at least annually. This should be of two or more weeks' duration if at all possible, as it takes longer than a week for the average person to relax and recharge. If in doubt, remember that it is almost unheard of for someone on their death bed to say, "I wish I had spent more time at the office."

What You Put into Your Mind

Another factor you control is what you put into your mind. The importance of the mind in determining one's level of wellness was addressed previously, but few take care to protect and nourish their mind. The average person takes more care in deciding what to put into a trash can than in determining what is put into his or her mind. This can be demonstrated by recognizing that horror movies are one of the most popular genres and that songs with demeaning lyrics are widely purchased.

What goes into your mind has a direct physical effect on your body. Your body is designed to be slightly alkaline, that is to say non-acidic. Degenerative diseases and cancers are more likely to appear if the tissues of the body have been acidic over time. Emotions of anger, hostility, bitterness, and frustration cause the body to become acidic, and no amount of dietary and supplemental effort will reverse the acidity brought on by unhealthy thoughts and emotions. Chronic acidity will cause bones to lose minerals as the body uses them to neutralize acid and restore an alkaline state. This truth is described in Proverbs 17:22: "A merry heart promotes healing, but a broken spirit dries up the bones." (I am aware that most English translations read "A merry heart does good like medicine," but the Hebrew word translated 'medicine' does not refer to the use of drugs, but rather to healing, as in the use of a bandage on a wound.)

The term "datasphere" has been coined to represent a source of information. When considering the mind, input can come from two dataspheres: an external datasphere and an internal datasphere. Your external datasphere consists of many information sources, including family members, friends, teachers, government, religious institutions, the Internet, print media (newspapers, books, and magazines), and broadcast media (radio, television, and movies). Your internal datasphere consists of data you give yourself. The internal datasphere is comprised largely of one's interpretation of events.

Information entering the mind from either datasphere can be supportive of health or destructive of health. If you are receiving data from the external datasphere that says the economy is bad, the dollar is falling in value, and terrorist attacks are on the rise, you may begin to feel helpless and, since you believe you lack control, emotions of fear and frustration will rise. If you are receiving data from the external datasphere suggesting that you have the ability to succeed despite the overall economic situation, you will experience positive emotions such as joy and hope. If your response to a challenge is "I'm an idiot!", "Circumstances are beyond my control!", or "I can't do anything right!", your internal datasphere is giving messages that will cause you further anxiety and frustration. If, on the other hand, you tell yourself "I'm intelligent!", "I control how I react to the circumstances that surround me!", or "I can make wise choices in life!", you are empowering yourself to take control of your situation, including your personal health challenges.

Since you cannot completely control your external datasphere, it is important that you critically examine the messages you are receiving from it. This is particularly true regarding messages that come through entertainment vehicles. It is important to approach amusements with caution, lest damaging messages creep in without you consciously being aware of them.

To muse means to be involved in deep thought. Since the prefix "a" means "without," to amuse means to be without deep thought. An amusement is an opportunity to inject messages while an individual is not thinking deeply. That is why *Webster's Ninth New Collegiate Dictionary* defines amuse as "To divert one's attention so as to deceive." When reading comic strips, watching movies, or watching television, begin to question the message behind the façade.

I once saw a cartoon that showed Moses coming down Mt. Sinai carrying two stone tablets. The caption read, "And don't forget to come back every ten years for updates. Times change, you know."[130] Some messages behind the "amusing" cartoon were that the Ten Commandments are outdated, that values are relative, and that morals change with the times.

Some of the subliminal messages in nearly all contemporary television sitcoms are that all men are buffoons, Christianity is absurd, marriage has failed as an institution, and it is normal to have sex early in life, as often as possible, with as many partners as possible. All of these messages detract from a person's ability to achieve and maintain optimum health.

The dominant messages of the external datasphere are that you are powerless, external forces beyond your control determine what your life will be like, and that your level of wellness is a matter of chance. What you allow into your mind from the external datasphere provides most of the resources of your internal datasphere. It is therefore important to choose your data sources wisely. You can exercise a great deal of control over your external datasphere, and you have total control over your internal datasphere.

Controlling your external datasphere means choosing the right friends, choosing information sources carefully, selecting encouraging reading material, eliminating most radio and television programming, and being selective when surfing the Internet. Controlling your internal datasphere means challenging the messages you give yourself and choosing wisely how you interpret events in your life. Screen messages, selecting those that are beneficial and reinforcing them. Avoid sources of destructive communications and add sources of constructive messages. When you control what enters your mind, you control your life.

I once met with a young woman who was frustrated and depressed. While looking for a source of her current condition, I learned that she had developed a very successful network marketing business that had collapsed when the company changed its compensation plan. She felt that she had betrayed her customers and misled those who had chosen to enter the business with her. She was unable to move forward because she feared hurting other people in the process.

The act of the company changing its compensation plan did not cause her depression and inability to move forward in a new direction. The company's action was simply an event. What had triggered her depression was the interpretation she had chosen to apply to that event (that she was a bad person for introducing people to the company's products and income-generating potential).

I challenged the interpretation she had put on the event. "Did you ever misrepresent the facts when you spoke to people about your products?" I asked. She said no. "Did anyone benefit from using the products?" I inquired. Her face lit up as she told about how many people had noted a significant improvement in their health while using the products. "Did you ever mislead anyone about how much income they could generate?" I questioned. She said that she had always been up front with people about the income potential. Finally, I asked if anyone who had decided to start their own business had earned any money. Again her face lit up as she told stories of how people had earned money that had significantly improved their financial picture.

"So," I suggested, "you helped a lot of people improve their health and you showed others how to strengthen their finances. Did you have any input into the company's decision to change their compensation plan?" She admitted that the changes had come as a complete surprise to her.

"Do you really believe that you were personally responsible for hurting anyone?" I challenged her to consider. As she reanalyzed what had transpired, she changed her interpretation of the event. No, she had been completely honest in all her dealings. She had helped people physically and financially. She had done nothing to harm anyone. Her depression lifted immediately. Within a month she had launched a new business, at which she has become very successful.

How You Nourish Your Spirit

The final factor you control that determines your level of wellness is how you nourish your spirit. One of the greatest examples of someone who constantly nourished his spirit was Nicolas Herman. He was born in early seventeenth-century France. He had no formal education and served for a time as a footman and soldier. He described himself as "a great awkward fellow who broke everything."[131] He entered a monastery in mid-life, where he was not considered worthy to take part in the theological discussions and so was assigned to the kitchen.

Ironically, none of the worthy brothers is remembered today. Nicolas Herman, however, is known worldwide as Brother Lawrence, author of "The Practice of the Presence of God." Brother Lawrence is recognized as a model of consistency, for he wrote, "The time of business does not with me differ from the time of prayer; and in the noise and clatter of my kitchen, while several persons are at the same time calling for different things, I possess God in as great tranquility as if I were upon my knees at the blessed sacrament."[132] He died at the age of eighty, full of love and honored by all.

Signs of a malnourished spirit include loss of the zest of living, a lack of dreams, and abandonment of hope. A malnourished spirit is seeking the answers to three fundamental questions of spiritual identity, without which it cannot thrive. The three questions are "Who am I?", "Why am I here?", and "Where am I going?"

The question "Who am I?" defines one's personal identity. You may define yourself by your occupation, your educational background, your position in society, your membership in various organizations, or your interpersonal relationships. While these can provide excellent answers to the question, each of them has the potential of being lost. You may lose your job or retire, you may lose your position in society, you may no longer qualify to be a member of a particular organization, and a close friend or family member may die.

How you define your identity will depend a great deal on how well you understand who you really are. You are more than a mass of aging tissue that is quickly passing away. You have a soul and a spirit that will survive long after your physical body has decomposed. I have chosen to define myself as a spiritual being, a child of God, an identity that cannot be lost, but will survive intact throughout eternity.

The question "Why Am I Here?" defines your life purpose. You may chose to say that your purpose is to earn a living, to build a business, to raise a family, to be of service to others, or to live life to the fullest. These too are excellent answers, but once again, they are subject to change. You may lose your ability to earn a living, your business may fail, your children may leave, and you may someday lose your ability to enjoy life to the fullest extent. My answer to the question is that I am here to do what God asks of me, and to show myself worthy of greater responsibility when I move from this life to the next. His calling may change over time, but my purpose will remain firm.

The answer to the question "Where am I going?" touches the heart of existence. It encompasses your goals and dreams and defines your vision. Most people have lost the ability to dream. I believe that is what makes them crabby. I have never personally gone crabbing, but I have been told that one need only catch two crabs to be able to keep them in a bucket. If a solitary crab is placed in a bucket it will crawl out. If two or more are present, however, as soon as one begins to crawl out the others pull it back down. Beware of crabby people. They will destroy your dreams and pull you down to their level.

Earlier I mentioned my experience with Brian Klemmer. Brian says that when he first began to work in the arena of personal development his boss told Brian that he was expected to write a life plan. Brian kept procrastinating until he was sent home and told not to return until his life plan was completed. Brian developed what he considered an aggressive plan for his life on earth. When he presented it to his boss, however, the man looked at it and asked, "That's it? You can't plan any farther than fifty years in the future?" Brian had been limited by thinking only of his *physical* existence. His mentor reminded Brian that he was a spiritual being living temporarily in a physical body.

The death of the physical body is not the end of one's life; it is simply the beginning of a new and exciting phase of existence. The Apostle Paul understood this well, for at one point he saw Paradise. Writing of his experience he says, "I know a man in Christ who fourteen years ago—whether in the body I do not know, or whether out of the body I do not know, God knows—such a one was caught up to the third heaven. And I know such a man—whether in the body or out of the body I do not know, God knows—how he was caught up into Paradise and heard inexpressible words, which it is not lawful for a man to utter."[133] This explains how he knew that physical death is not the end of one's life, "what you sow is not made alive unless it dies . . . So also is the resurrection of the dead. The body is sown in corruption, it is raised in incorruption. It is sown in dishonor, it is raised in glory. It is sown in weakness, it is raised in power. It is sown a natural body, it is raised a spiritual body. There is a natural body, and there is a spiritual body."[134]

Paul stated that he did not know whether his glimpse of heaven was a vision or an out of the body experience. I believe it was the latter, for it is reported in the book of Acts that Paul was stoned in the city of Lystra, dragged out of the city, and left for dead.[135] It is unlikely that those who stoned him and drug him out of the city would have failed to notice if he had still been breathing. It is even more implausible that Paul, after being stoned to the point of appearing to be dead, could have stood up, walked back into the city, and continued on his journey the following day. I believe that Paul was stoned to death, was given a glimpse of life after physical death, and then miraculously brought back to life to continue his work on earth.

Many people become too concerned with the activities and demands of daily life on earth to consider that there is life beyond the grave. When that truth is grasped, however, it changes one's perspective. If I believe that I die with my body my focus will be solely on what I can accomplish during my physical existence on earth. If I realize that greater opportunities await me when I leave my physical body behind, I will focus less on the acquisition of material goods and more on the cultivation of relationships that I will cherish throughout eternity.

I do not subscribe to the popular notion that life after death consists of sitting on a cloud playing a harp. The future I read about in the Bible is far more exciting. I am told that I will not only have access to the dimension we call heaven, but that I will have a position of responsibility on a new earth. "(You) have made us kings and priests to our God; And we shall reign on the earth."[136]

Where am I going? I am going to be reunited with many of the people I have loved here on earth and spend eternity with them in God's presence. In addition, I am striving to run a good race here on earth so that when I leave my physical body I will hear the words, "'Well done, good and faithful servant; you were faithful over a few things, I will make you ruler over many things. Enter into the joy of your lord.'"[137]

How about you? Do you have a life plan? If you do, how far does it extend into the future? Are you content to settle for what you can accomplish in the time you exist in your physical body, or do you want to play a bigger game? If you do, deliberately nourish your spirit moment by moment and day by day.

One of the ways you can nourish your spirit is by observing the beauty that surrounds you. Seeing a dry leaf in the snow inspired Brother Lawrence to commit himself to the practice of God's presence with him. Enjoy the arts, which are sources of inspiration that speak to the spirit. These include music, visual arts, dance, prose, poetry, and oratory. Embrace your fellow creatures, not only plants and animals, but most importantly other people. Above all, like Brother Lawrence, practice the presence of God in your life.

He is the Great Physician, the source of all healing. He is available anytime and anywhere. He does not charge for His services, and all who seek Him find Him. He is worth finding, for He has promised that He will give you the desires of your heart!

Chapter 16

Putting It All Together – A Basic Wellness Regimen

Heal me, O LORD, and I shall be healed; Save me, and I shall be saved,
For You are my praise.
– Jeremiah 17:14

In the preceding chapters I have related what I have learned about the mechanisms of disease and aging over a period of over forty years. It may at first seem overwhelming to consider all of the factors needed to experience optimum wellness. The good news is that it is usually not necessary to make dramatic changes in your lifestyle to achieve major benefits. Implement changes in a manner that makes sense to you, changes that you are willing to adopt over the long run. When one beneficial practice becomes a comfortable part of your daily routine, institute another. Remember that there is a continuum between sickness and wellness and that the goal is to be moving toward wellness rather than sliding toward sickness over time.

Concentrate on the Basics

The start of a new season in sports is an exciting time for fans and players alike. It brings a sense that the slate is clean and that there is an opportunity to begin anew. It is often a time of reflection and resolving to do better.

As teams arrive in training camp for their preseason workouts, they inevitably go back to the basics. The focus is not so much on developing new strategies as it is on conditioning and on developing the skills necessary to play well. Depending upon the sport, these may include running, throwing, catching, blocking, tackling, dribbling, or shooting.

The same should be true for each of us as we resolve to do better. No matter what aspect of our life we are hoping to improve, it is always best to go back to the basics. This is particularly true in improving our state of wellness.

I do not believe in the magic bullet approach to health; there is no single supplement that will restore health if the basics are ignored. My protocols, which are specific to various health challenges, always build off of the basics. When the basics are ignored, the outcome is often less than desired.

I see examples of this regularly. A short time ago, an individual who was fighting depression called me to report his progress. I had recommended that he follow a basic wellness regimen and add 5-HTP, the last building block needed in the manufacture of seratonin. He had done well for a time, but he now reported that symptoms of depression were returning. I asked what had changed. He was under no undue stress. He was still taking the 5-HTP. He had run out of his broad-spectrum vitamin/mineral/amino acid supplement several weeks before, he admitted, and had not bothered to refill it.

I was not surprised that his symptoms had returned, for 5-HTP does not automatically turn into seratonin when it enters the body. The vitamin and mineral nutrients that are required for its conversion to seratonin must also be present. As the level of those substances fell, the process stalled, and the young man's symptoms of seratonin deficiency returned.

Drinking pure water is the first wellness basic. The body's need for water is so great that entire books have been written on the subject. It is required for nearly all life processes. Water is second only to the oxygen we breathe as the substance most necessary to maintain life. It is possible to survive for weeks without food, but death will occur within days if water is unavailable. I discussed the characteristics of water when I wrote of treating the body like a palace. I now remind you that the most accurate indicator of adequate hydration is the ability to pass pale urine every few hours. Getting into the habit of drinking sixteen ounces of water over a fifteen minute period mid-morning and mid-afternoon can be helpful in assuring adequate hydration and improving elimination of wastes from the body.

Breathing clean air is as important as drinking pure water. If you are a nonsmoker, don't start, and if you are a smoker, do whatever is necessary to stop. It is difficult to imagine anything more damaging to optimum health than inhaling hot, noxious gases on a regular basis. Remember that the indoor air quality in most American homes is worse than the outdoor air quality in large U.S. cities. Steps should be taken to correct this situation, beginning with changing filters in heating and air conditioning systems regularly.

Get your body moving and keep it moving for twenty to thirty minutes three to five times a week. Remember that you are pushing too hard too soon if you cannot last for thirty minutes without stopping, if you cannot talk out loud while you are performing the activity, or if you feel stiff and sore the next day.

Observe the rules for healthy eating. Keep your diet colorful. Eat only items that would remain edible at room temperature. Stick to unrefined foods. Avoid refined sugars and flours. Seek out whole grain foods. Avoid additives, preservatives and artificial sweeteners. Include vegetable oils in salad dressings or salsas. Include legumes (beans, peas). Keep meat portions small by viewing meats, fish and poultry as items that provide distinctive flavors to your meals rather than as the "main course" and using the size of the palm of your hand or the size of a standard deck of playing cards to estimate the appropriate serving size. Finally, vary the foods you eat over the course of each week.

Limit your exposure to toxic chemicals. Use a shower filter and, if bathing, fill the tub through the filter. Use nontoxic personal care items (shampoo and conditioner, soaps, toothpaste, deodorant, sunscreen, cosmetics, etc.) and nontoxic cleaning agents.

Provide electromagnetic support for your body and place electromagnetic shielding appliances on cellular and portable telephones. Remember that what you can't see *can* kill you.

Address the biochemical mechanisms of aging and disease development. Provide a broad-spectrum nutritional supplement as a base upon which to build nutritional support. Take a plant-based oligoproanthocyanidin (OPC) supplement to protect your body tissues from free radical damage. Supplement omega-3 fatty acids to give your body the raw materials needed to manufacture anti-inflammatory compounds. Check your homocysteine level and if it is greater than seven micromoles/liter, add a comprehensive support for the methylation process. As you enter your fifties add a mitochondrial support to prevent age-related mitochondrial decline.

Have a computer system check run at least annually. Do this sooner if symptoms of illness appear or you encounter a period of significant physical or emotional stress.

Provide mind supplements as well. Break the "news" habit; listen to uplifting messages and read good books.

Finally, and most importantly, develop a relationship with your Creator. Neglect this and nothing else matters. You are first and foremost a spiritual being. Your ultimate fate will be determined in the spiritual, not the material realm. Jesus taught, "I have come that they may have life, and that they may have it more abundantly." I do not believe that He was making a "pie in the sky by and by when I die to go to Heaven" offer, but stating the fact that abundant living is possible on earth for those who desire it. I encourage you to start living an abundant life in the here and now. You will never regret your decision.

Epilogue

The Importance of Taking Action

But be doers of the word, and not hearers only, deceiving yourselves.
– James 1:22

As stated at the outset, you are fearfully and wonderfully made. Your body contains incredible healing mechanisms capable of dealing with health challenges, but they must be supported to function effectively. Building health by design does not require the use of costly, high-tech devices or procedures. It does require a conscientious effort to provide support and protection to your body to minimize the challenges it will face and to maximize its ability to respond quickly and effectively when challenges do occur.

How long any specific individual will live depends upon many factors, some of which are genetically determined. Regardless of your genetic makeup, however, your life expectancy will be increased by building health by design. More significantly, you will enjoy a much higher quality of life throughout your time on this earth.

Taking small steps toward improved health can often result in major rewards. When all known mechanisms of aging and disease development are addressed, miracles can happen. I know, because I regularly see people who experience what I would have considered miraculous recoveries in my former standard medical practice. In actuality, they are miracles—miracles of the body's marvelous and intelligent design.

I am currently sixty-three years young. If I were to die tomorrow, someone might say that building my health by design had been of no benefit to me, since I had not lived to an advanced age. I am convinced, however, that I have already added ten productive years to my life. More important to me is the fact that I feel much better, have more energy, and am able to enjoy life to a much greater extent than I did when I was forty. The constant fatigue, muscle tenderness, joint pain, and foggy headedness that characterized my life in my early forties are now only distant and fading memories.

My father, who was physically active, ate a decent diet, and did not use tobacco products, died suddenly of a heart attack at the age of fifty-four. My brother experienced a heart attack at the age of forty-five. Thankfully, he survived. At a reunion of my father's side of my family, I found it nearly impossible to find a male cousin over the age of fifty who had not had a heart attack or surgical repair of a coronary artery.

I am not "lucky" to have avoided coronary artery disease. I have the same genetic predisposition to a heart attack as that of my relatives. Pictures of me in my early forties reveal a pasty gray complexion consistent with someone in the process of committing suicide on the installment plan. If I had not learned that atherosclerosis develops not because of high cholesterol levels, but because of arterial inflammation and oxidative damage to LDL cholesterol, and if I had not taken action to reduce inflammation and stop free radical damage, I would not be alive today.

You now have the knowledge needed to optimize your health and maximize your life. Having knowledge, however, is not enough. To achieve success you must act on what you know. I have spoken with other physicians who admit that oxidized LDL cholesterol, not total or normal LDL cholesterol, is a key factor in arterial plaque development. Nevertheless, they continue to prescribe cholesterol-lowering medications rather than recommending antioxidant and anti-inflammatory supports. I have explained the mechanism of plaque buildup to individuals in my office and to groups of people on radio, television, and in seminars and workshops. Sadly, many admit that while what they have learned makes sense, they are not willing to act on the information because they fear it will upset their personal physician.

You hold the keys that open the doors to optimum wellness. You can choose to use them to open those doors, or you can choose to toss the keys in a drawer where you can find them in case they are needed at some future time. Keep in mind, however, that the sooner action is taken, the greater is the chance for success. In the words of Poor Richard, "An ounce of prevention is worth a pound of cure." It is also considerably less expensive.

Knowledge is only beneficial if it leads to action. Good intentions are admirable, but unless they are acted upon they are of no benefit. An old riddle drives the point home. Ten frogs were sitting on a log. One of them decided to jump. How many frogs are still on the log?

The correct answer is ten. Deciding to do something is not the same as actually doing it. I hope that you *decide* to begin building your health by design, but even more I hope that you *do* begin to build your health by design. I hope that you begin living abundantly today and that you continue to do so throughout eternity. The Creator who designed your body desires nothing less!

Appendix A
A Guide to Nutritional Supplementation

I did not write *Building Health by Design* to promote a particular company or product line. The message it contains is far too important to limit it in that way. It is my intent that people who are already using nutritional products that address the various mechanisms of premature aging and disease continue to do so. I do not wish to convert those individuals to "my brand," nor do I wish customers of reputable companies to change their purchasing habits.

The leading criticism of those who reviewed the manuscript prior to publication, however, was that I had not included specific product recommendations for individuals who are not familiar with nutritional supplementation. I therefore chose to include specific examples in Appendix B: A Basic Wellness Regimen.

How to Determine the Quality of Nutritional Supplements

The nutritional supplement industry is largely self-regulating. Many reputable companies produce high quality nutritional supports, but there are also companies that sell supplements that use inferior ingredients or do not contain the ingredients listed on the label. When I first began recommending nutritional supplements in the management of health challenges, I took a generic approach. I would, for example, suggest that the individual purchase St. John's wort at a local health food or discount store. As often as not, the person would return and report that their condition had not improved. At that point I faced an unanswerable question—had my assessment been incorrect and my recommendation invalid or had the patient simply purchased an inferior product? It was only after I began recommending that patients purchase products that I knew from my personal research were of high quality that I began to see consistent results. I do not demand that people stay on those products once a response has been achieved; they are welcome to purchase other brands at that point because they will know if the product is not producing the desired effect.

It is impossible for me to personally evaluate each manufacturer of nutritional supplements. I can, however, give you four questions to ask in determining whether or not appropriate steps are being taken to assure that the end product is of consistent quality.

1) Are all lots of raw materials checked for quality and purity before they are incorporated into any product? This is necessary for all ingredients, but it is especially important for herbal substances. If the dried and ground material being sold as milk thistle, which supports liver function, is actually common chickweed, the product that contains it will not provide the desired benefit.

2) Are the most bioavailable forms of the nutrients used? (Can the body effectively absorb and utilize the nutrient in the form provided?) For example, chelated forms of minerals such as calcium citrate or magnesium aspartate are absorbed and utilized much better than calcium carbonate or magnesium oxide. The effectiveness of a product can be impacted greatly by the form of a particular nutrient that is used in the formulation.

3) Does the manufacturer follow a pharmaceutical grade standard? This means that each serving of each product has exactly the same amount of nutrients as other servings in the lot and that the level of nutrients in a serving is what is stated on the label.

4) Is each lot of product tested for quality and purity before being released for sale? This assures that no contaminants have entered the product and that the nutrient levels are what they are said to be.

I use products from many different manufacturers in my practice, but my primary supplier is Vitality Laboratories in Reno, Nevada. They have been manufacturing nutritional products without compromising quality for over two decades, and I have worked personally with President Gary Paulsen for nearly a decade. I know that he will use the form of each nutrient I recommend when formulating a product, and I know that he will destroy a run of capsules if the lot does not meet specifications. The list in Appendix B features the MVP brand of nutritional supplements manufactured by Vitality Laboratories. It is the regimen I use personally, but I do not intend to imply that it is the only acceptable way of *Building Health by Design.*

Appendix B
A Basic Wellness Regimen

- Drink pure water
  - Drink only distilled or reverse osmosis filtered water. Reverse osmosis is preferred.
  - Drink enough to keep your urine pale. Thirst is not an efficient mechanism for maintaining adequate hydration.
  - Flush your system by drinking 16 ounces of water over a 15 minute time period mid-morning and mid-afternoon.
- Breathe clean air
  - Don't smoke.
  - Change or clean furnace filters regularly.
  - Use air purifiers in the home and office.
- Follow these rules for healthy eating
  - Keep your diet colorful.
  - Eat only items that would remain edible at room temperature.
  - Stick to unrefined foods.
    - Avoid refined sugars and flours. Seek out whole grain foods.
    - Avoid additives, preservatives and artificial sweeteners.
  - Include vegetable oils in salad dressings or salsas.
  - Include legumes (beans, peas).
  - Keep meat portions small.
    - View meats, fish and poultry as items that provide distinctive flavors to your meals rather than the "main course."
    - Use the size of the palm of your hand or the size of a standard deck of playing cards as the size of a serving.
  - Vary the foods you eat.
- Stay physically active
  - Get your body moving and keep it moving for 20-30 minutes at least every other day (3-5 times per week).

- You are pushing too hard too soon if:
  - You cannot last for 30 minutes without stopping.
  - You cannot talk out loud while you are doing the activity.
  - You feel stiff and sore the next day.
- Limit exposure to toxic chemicals
  - Use non-toxic personal care items (shampoo and conditioner, soaps, toothpaste, deodorant, sunscreen, cosmetics, etc.).
  - Use only non-toxic cleaning agents around the home and office.
  - Use a shower filter.
- Use electromagnetic protective devices
  - EP-2 pendant for personal protection
  - E-Dot to reduce cell phone radiation
- Take nutritional supplements
  - *Lifetime*—One tablet or two capsules per thirty pounds of body weight daily divided into two servings (with breakfast and with dinner). Formulated by Dr. Robert Preston, who recognized that over one hundred nutrients are needed by the body for daily maintenance and repair. Rather than asking patients to purchase multiple products, he chose to put all of the nutrients into one bottle. He called the product Lifetime because he believed that it contained the nutrients his body needed to remain healthy over the course of his lifetime. Lifetime provides a sound base of nutrients upon which to build. If someone chooses to take nothing but Lifetime I know they will tend to do well. Using mechanism specific supports will provide added protection.
  - *OPC 2000*—One capsule per fifty pounds of body weight twice daily. The combination of antioxidant nutrients in Lifetime and the grape seed and skin extracts in OPC 2000 provide excellent support for the body's antioxidant defense mechanism.
  - *Marine Lipids*—One capsule twice daily. Marine Lipids contain omega-3 fish oils that provide the raw materials the body needs to manufacture anti-inflammatory compounds.
  - *Panzymes* may be taken as needed to control inflammation. Conditions that end in "itis" are an indication for use of Panzymes. Four to six

capsules are taken two or three times daily, at least one hour before or two hours after eating.

- *HCY Formula*—Three to six capsules twice daily. I formulated HCY Formula to support the body's methylation mechanism. It contains the nutrients described in the chapter on methylation (*Support Your Local Handyman*). Need for HCY Formula is indicated by a homocysteine level greater than 7.2 mmol/L.

- *XTra Mile* or *Ochtane* (the same product is sold under two brand names)—One capsule two or three times daily. I formulated Xtra Mile/Ochtane to support the body's ability to utilize oxygen effectively to produce energy. It contains the nutrients described in the chapter on mitochondrial decline (*Put the Pedal to the Metal*) as supporting mitochondrial function.

- Provide mind supplements
  - Break the "news" habit.
  - Listen to uplifting tapes and read good books.
- Develop a relationship with your Creator
  - We are first and foremost spiritual beings.
  - Neglect this and nothing else matters.

Appendix C
Product Sources

Educational Articles and Support Protocols
http://www.drdalepeterson.com

Energy Protective Devices
http://www.shopemf.com

Nutritional Supplements
Maximum Vitality Partners
5350 Capital Court, Suite number 109
Reno, NV 89502
(800)423-8365
http://www.mvpontheweb.com/drpeterson

Water and Air Purification
Water and Air Essentials
1850 N. Greenville Ave., Suite 184
Richardson, Texas 75081
(800)964-4303
http://www.ewater.com/drpeterson

Notes

1. *Indoor Air Pollution: An Introduction for Health Professionals, U.S. Government Printing Office Publication No. 1994-523-217/81322. 1994.*

2. Ehlen, L.A., et al. "Acidic beverages increase the risk of in vitro tooth erosion." *Nutr Res.* 28(May 2008): 299–303.

3. Ludwig, D.S., K.E. Peterson, and S.L. Gortmaker. "Relation between consumption of sugar-sweetened drinks and childhood obesity: a prospective, observational analysis." *Lancet.* 357(Feb. 17 2001): 505–8.

4. Heaney, Robert P. and Karen Rafferty. "Carbonated beverages and urinary calcium excretion." *Am J. Clin Nutr.* 74(2001): 343–47.

5. Tucker, K.L, et al. "Colas, but not other carbonated beverages, are associated with low bone mineral density in older women: The Framingham Osteoporosis Study." *Am J Clin Nutr.* 84(Oct. 2006): 936–42.

6. Wyshak, G. "Teenaged girls, carbonated beverage consumption, and bone fractures." *Arch Pediatr Adolesc Med.* 154(2000): 610–13.

7. Saldana, T.M., et al. "Carbonated Beverages and Chronic Kidney Disease." *Epidemiology.* 18(Jul. 2007): 501–6.

8. Kronberger, Hans, and Siegbert Lattacher. *On the Track of Water's Secret - from Victor Schauberger to Johann Grander.* Vienna: Uranus, 1995.

9. Campbell, T. Colin. *The China Study.* BenBella Books, 2005.

10. Rahman, I., and W. MacNee. "Role of antioxidants in smoking-induced lung disease." *Free Rad Biol Med.* 21(1996): 669–81.

11. Okuyama, H. "Need to change the direction of cholesterol-related medication—a problem of great urgency." *Yakugaku Zasshi.* 125(Nov. 2005): 833–52.

12. Singh, G. "Recent Considerations in Nonsteroidal Anti-Inflammatory Drug Gastropathy." *Am J Med.* 105(Jul. 27, 1998)(1B): 31S–38S.

13. Loes, Michael, and David Steinman. *The Aspirin Alternative.* Topanga, CA: Freedom Press, 2001.

14. Dzhak, F.W. "Use of Wobenzym in the Treatment of Muscle Damage in Athletes." Presented at Second Russian Symposium on Oral Enzyme Therapy, St. Petersburg, Russia, 1996. 65–67.

15. Loes, op. cit. 125–27.

16. Ibid. 156–57.

17. Salles-Montaudon, N., et al. "Prevalence and mechanisms of hyperhomocysteinemia in elderly hospitalized patients." *J Nutr Health Aging.* 7(2003)(2): 111–16.

18. Ventura, P., et al. "Hyperhomocysteinemia and related factors in 600 hospitalized elderly subjects." *Metabolism.* 50(Dec. 2001): 1466–71.

19. Asanuma, Y., et al. "Premature coronary-artery atherosclerosis in systemic lupus erythematosis." *N Engl J Med.* 349 (Dec. 18, 2003): 2407–15.

20. Pueschel, S.M., W.Y. Craig, and J.E. Haddow. "Lipids and lipoproteins in persons with Down's syndrome." *J Intellect Disabil Res.* 36(4)(Aug. 1992): 365–69.

21. "American Heart Association position statement on homocysteine." American Heart Association website. http://www.americanheart.org. Aug. 2010.

22. McCaddon, A., et al. "Total serum homocysteine in senile dementia of Alzheimer type." *Int J Geriatr Psychiatry.* 13(Apr. 1998): 235–39.

23. Joosten, E., et al. "Is metabolic evidence for vitamin B-12 and folate deficiency more frequent in elderly patients with Alzheimer's disease?" *J Gerontol A Biol Sci Med Sci.* 52(2)(Mar. 1997): M76–79.

24. Verhoef, P., et. al. "Homocysteine Metabolism and risk of myocardial infarction: relation with vitamins B6, B12, and folate." *Am J Epidemiol.* 143(May 1, 1996): 845–59.

25. Humphrey, L.L., et al. "Homocysteine level and coronary heart disease incidence: a systematic review and meta-analysis." *Mayo Clin Proc.* 83(Nov. 2008): 1203–12.

26. Rinehart, J.F., and L.D. Greenberg. "Arteriosclerotic lesions in pyridoxine-deficient monkeys." *Fed. Proc.* 7(1948): 278.

27. Capretti, G., and B. Magnani. "Vitamin B6 and experimental cholesterol atherosclerosis." *G Clin Med.* 32(Apr. 1951): 417–24.

28. McCully, K.S. "Vascular pathology of homocysteinemia: Implications for the pathogenesis of arteriosclerosis." *Amer J Path.* 56(1969): 111–28.

29. Hattersley, J. "Acquired Atherosclerosis: Theories of Causation, Novel Therapies." *Journal of Orthomolecular Medicine.* 6(2)(1991): 83–98.

30. Ellis, J.M., and K.S. McCully. "Prevention of myocardial infarction by vitamin B6." *Res Commun Mol Pathol Pharmacol.* 89(2)(Aug. 1995): 208–20.

31. Israelsson, B., L.E. Brattström, and B.L. Hultberg. "Homocysteine and myocardial infarction." *Atherosclerosis.* 71(2-3)(Jun. 1988): 227–33.

32. Fortin, L.J., and J. Genest, Jr. "Measurement of homocyst(e)ine in the prediction of arteriosclerosis." *Clin Biochem.* 28(1995): 155–62.

33. Kang, S.S., P.W. Wong, and M. Norusis. "Homocysteinemia due to folate deficiency." *Metabolism.* 36(May 1987): 458–62.

34. Seller, M.J. "Vitamins, folic acid and the cause and prevention of neural tube defects." *Ciba Found Symp.* 181(1994): 161–73; discussion 173–79.

35. Forman, R., et al. "Folic acid and prevention of neural tube defects: a study of Canadian mothers of infants with spina bifida." *Clin Invest Med.* 19(3)(Jun. 1996): 195–201.

36. Duerre, J.A., and J.C. Wallwork. "Methionine metabolism in isolated perfused livers from rats fed on zinc-deficient and restricted diets." *Br J Nutr.* 56(2)(Sep. 1986): 395–405.

37. Millian, N.S., and T.A. Garrow. "Human betaine-homocysteine methyltransferase is a zinc metalloenzyme." *Arch Biochem Biophys.* 356(Aug. 1, 1998): 93–98.

38. Anderson, T.W. "Water hardness, magnesium and ischemic heart disease." *Nova Scotia Med Bull.* 56(1977): 58–61.

39. Howard, J.M. "Magnesium Deficiency in Peripheral Vascular Disease." *Journal of Nutritional and Environmental Medicine.* 1(1)(1990): 39–49.

40. McGregor, D.O., et al. "Betaine supplementation decreases post-methionine hyperhomocysteinemia in chronic renal failure." *Kidney Int.* 61(Mar. 2002): 1040–46.

41. Olthof, M.R., and P. Verhoef. "Effects of betaine intake on plasma homocysteine concentrations and consequences for health." *Curr Drug Metab.* 6(1)(Feb. 2005): 15–22.

42. Bostom, A.G., et al. "Lack of effect of oral N-acetylcysteine on the acute dialysis-related lowering of total plasma homocysteine in hemodialysis patients." *Atherosclerosis.* 120(Feb. 1996): 241–44.

43. Ventura, P., et al. "Urinary and plasma homocysteine and cysteine levels during prolonged oral N-acetylcysteine therapy." *Pharmacology.* 68(2)(Jun. 2003): 105–14.

44. Milani, R.V., and C.J. Lavie. "Homocysteine: the Rubik's cube of cardiovascular risk factors." *Mayo Clin Proc.* 83(Nov. 2008): 1200–02.

45. Folkers, K., P. Langsioen, and P.H. Langsioen. "Therapy with coenzyme Q10 of patients in heart failure who are eligible or ineligible for a transplant." *Biochem Biophys Res Commun.* 182(Jan. 15, 1992): 247–53.

46. Goa, K.L., and R.N. Brogden. "l-Carnitine. A preliminary review of its pharmacokinetics, and its therapeutic use in ischaemic cardiac disease and primary and secondary carnitine deficiencies in relationship to its role in fatty acid metabolism." *Drugs.* 34(1)(Jul. 1987): 1-24.

47. Oguro, H., et al. "Successful treatment with succinate in a patient with MELAS." *Intern Med.* 43(May 2004): 427–31.

48. Weinberg, J.M., et al. "Anaerobic and aerobic pathways for salvage of proximal tubules from hypoxia-induced mitochondrial injury." *Am J Physiol Renal Physiol.* 279(5)(Nov. 2000): F927–43.

49. Hagen, T.M., et al. "Feeding acetyl-L-carnitine and lipoic acid to old rats significantly improves metabolic function while decreasing oxidative stress." *Proc Natl Acad Sci USA.* 99(Feb. 19, 2002): 1870–75. Erratum in: *Proc Natl Acad Sci USA.* 99(10)(May 14, 2002): 7184.

50. Hagen, T.M., et al. "(R)-alpha-lipoic acid-supplemented old rats have improved mitochondrial function, decreased oxidative damage, and increased metabolic rate." *FASEB J.* 13(Feb. 1999): 411–18.

51. **Scopesi, F., et al.** "Dietary Nucleotide Supplementation Raises Erythrocyte 2,3-Diphosphoglycerate Concentration in Neonatal Rats." *Journal of Nutrition.* 129(1999): 662–65.

52. Chen, P., et al. "Inosine induces axonal rewiring and improves behavioral outcome after stroke." *Proc Natl Acad Sci USA.* 99(13)(Jun. 25, 2002): 9031–36.

53. Markowitz, C.E., et al. "The treatment of multiple sclerosis with inosine." *J Altern Complement Med.* 15(Jun. 2009): 619–25.

54. Grattagliano, I., et al. "Effect of dietary restriction and N-acetylcysteine supplementation on intestinal mucosa and liver mitochondrial redox status and function in aged rats." *Exp Gerontol.* 39(Sep. 2004): 1323–32.

55. SEER Cancer Statistics Review 1975 – 2007. National Cancer Institute. Devcan Version 6.5.0 (June 2010).

56. Rong-Gong, L. "Alzheimer's now a top killer in L.A. County." *Los Angeles Times*. November 16, 2006.

57. Brown, R.T., et al. "Prevalence and assessment of attention-deficit/hyperactivity disorder in primary care settings." *Pediatrics*. 107(Mar. 2001): E43.

58. Froehlich, T.E., et al. "Prevalence, Recognition, and Treatment of Attention-Deficit/Hyperactivity Disorder in a National Sample of US Children." *Arch Pediatr Adolesc Med*. 161(9)(2007): 857–64.

59. "Consensus Document on Fibromyalgia: The Copenhagen Declaration." *Journal of Musculoskeletal Pain*. 2(3): 295–312.

60. Lawrence, R.C., et al. "National Arthritis Work Group Estimates of the prevalence of arthritis and other rheumatic conditions in the United States. Part II." *Arthritis Rheum*. 58(2008): 26–35.

61. "Your guide to healthy sleep." NHLBI Health Information Center. NIH Publication No. 06–5800. April 2006.

62. Berger, K., and T. Kurth. "RLS epidemiology, frequencies, risk factors and methods in population studies." *Mov Disord*. 22(suppl 18)(2007): S420–S423.

63. Schlender, Shelly. Radio Interview with Jerry Phillips, August 20, 2006. KGNU Radio archives.

64. *Microwave News*. 24(4)(July 2006).

65. Cribb, R., and T. Hamilton. "Is her cell phone safe?" *Toronto Star*. July 10, 2005.

66. Harrill, R. "Wake up call." *University of Washington Alumni Magazine*. Columns, March 2005.

67. Volkradt, W. "Are Microwaves faced with a Fiasco similar to that experienced by Nuclear Energy?" *Wetter-Boden-Mensch*. April 1991.

68. "'Radiation Research' and the cult of negative results." *Microwave News*. 26(4)(July 2006).

69. Utteridge, T.D., et al. "Long-term exposure of E-mu-Pim1 transgenic mice to 898.4 MHz microwaves does not increase lymphoma incidence." *Radiat Res*. 158(3)(Sep. 2002): 357–64.

70. Harst, W., J. Kuhn, and H. Stever. "Can Electromagnetic Exposure Cause a Change in Behaviour? Studying Possible Non-Thermal Influences on Honey Bees – An Approach within the Framework of Educational Informatics." *Acta Systemica*. 6(1)(2006): 1–6.

71. Dambeck, H. "Debunking a new myth: Mobile Phones and Dying Bees." *Der Spiegel Online*. April 18, 2007. http://www.spiegel.de/international/ world/0,1518,477804,00.html.

72. Sharma, Ved Parkash, and Neelima R. Kumar. "Changes in honeybee behaviour and biology under the influence of cellphone radiations." *Current Science*. 98(May 25, 2010).

73. Selvin, S., J. Schulman, and D.W. Merrill. "Distance and risk measures for the analysis of spatial data: a study of childhood cancers." *Soc Sci Med*. 34(7)(Apr. 1992): 769–77.

74. Cherry, N. "Childhood cancer incidence in the vicinity of the Sutro Tower, San Francisco." Environmental Management and Design Division, Lincoln University, Canterbury, New Zealand. May 6, 2000.

75. Dolk, H., et al. 'Cancer incidence near radio and television transmitters in Great Britain. I. Sutton Coldfield transmitter." *Am J Epidemiol*. 1459(Jan. 1, 1997): 1–9.

76. Hocking, B., et al. 'Cancer incidence and mortality and proximity to TV towers." *Med J Aust*. 165(11-12)(Dec. 1996): 601–05.

77. Michelozzi, P., et al. "Leukemia mortality and incidence of infantile leukemia near the Vatican Radio Station of Rome." *Epidemiol Prev*. 25(6)(Nov.-Dec. 2001): 249–55.

78. Hallberg, O., and O. Johansson. "Malignant melanoma of the skin - not a sunshine story!" *Med Sci Monit*. 10(2004): CR336–40.

79. Hallberg, O., and O. Johansson. "Cancer trends during the twentieth century." *ACNEM Journal*. 21(1)(April 2002): 3–8.

80. Coray, R., et al. "NIR Exposure of Salzburg." Federal Office of Communications. February 2002.

81. Hardell, L., M. Carlberg, and Mild K. Hansson. "Pooled analysis of two case-control studies on the use of cellular and cordless telephones and the risk of benign brain tumours diagnosed during 1997-2003." *Int J Oncol*. 28(Feb. 2006): 509–18.

82. Hepworth, S.J., et al. "Mobile phone use and risk of glioma in adults: case-control study." *BMJ*. 332(7546)(Apr. 15, 2006): 883–87.

83. Lai, H., and N.P. Singh. "Acute low-intensity microwave exposure increases DNA single-strand breaks in rat brain cells." *Bioelectromagnetics*. 16(3)(1995): 207–10.

84. Phillips, J., et al. "DNA Damage in Molt-4 T-lymphoblastoid cells exposed to cellular telephone radiofrequency fields in vitro." *Bioelectrochemistry and Bioenergetics.* 45(1)(March 1998): 103–10.

85. Schlender, loc. cit.

86. Diem, E., et. al. "Non-thermal DNA breakage by mobile-phone radiation (1800 MHz) in human fibroblasts and in transformed GFSH-R17 rat granulosa cells in vitro." *Mutat Res.* 583(2)(Jun. 6, 2005): 178–83.

87. Zhang, D.Y., et al. "Effects of GSM 1800 MHz radiofrequency electromagnetic fields on DNA damage in Chinese hamster lung cells." *Zhonghua Yu Fang Yi Xue Za Zhi.* 40(3)(May 2006): 149–52.

88. Workshop on possible biological and health effects of RF electromagnetic fields. Vienna EMF-Resolution. Project Team: Mobile Phones and Health. Symposium, University of Vienna, Austria. October 25-28, 1998.

89. International Conference on Cell Tower Siting: Linking Science and Public Health. Salzburg, June 7-8, 2000.

90. Stewart, Sir William (Chairman). "*Mobile Phones and Health: A report from the Independent Expert Group on Mobile Phones.*" Chilton, IEGMP Secretariat (May 2000).

91. "Catania Resolution 2002." *Electromagnetic Biology and Medicine.* 25(4)(Dec. 2006): 201–02.

92. "Mobile Phones and Health 2004: Report by Stewart/National Radiological Protection Board, United Kingdom, NRPB." 15(5).

93. "Benevento Resolution." *Electromagnetic Biology and Medicine.* 25(2006): 197–200.

94. Evans, N., ed. *State of the evidence: What Is the Connection Between the Environment and Breast Cancer?* 4th ed. San Francisco: Breast Cancer Fund, 2006.

95. Li, C.Y., and F.C. Sung. "Association between occupational exposure to power frequency electromagnetic fields and amyotrophic lateral sclerosis: a review." *Am J Ind Med.* 43(2)(Feb. 2003): 212–20.

96. Qiu, C., et al. "Occupational exposure to electromagnetic fields and risk of Alzheimer's disease." *Epidemiology.* 15(6)(Nov. 2004): 687–94.

97. Noonan, C.W., et al. "Occupational exposure to magnetic fields in case-referent studies of neurodegenerative diseases." *Scand J Work Environ Health.* 28(1)(Feb. 2002): 42–48.

98. Persson, B.R., et al. "Increased permeability of the blood-brain barrier induced by magnetic and electromagnetic fields." *Ann N Y Acad Sci.* 649(Mar. 31, 1992): 356–58.

99. Salford, L.G., et al. "Nerve cell damage in mammalian brain after exposure to microwaves from GSM mobile phones." *Environ Health Perspect.* 111(7)(Jun. 2003): 881–83.

100. de Pomerai, D.I., et al. "Microwave radiation can alter protein conformation without bulk heating." *FEBS Lett.* 543(1-3)(May 22, 2003): 93–97.

101. Mancinelli, F., et al. "Non-thermal effects of electromagnetic fields at mobile phone frequency on the refolding of an intracellular protein: myoglobin." *J Cell Biochem.* 93(1)(Sep. 1, 2004: 188–96.

102. Ilhan, A., et al. "Ginkgo biloba prevents mobile phone-induced oxidative stress in rat brain." *Clin Chim Acta.* 340(1-2)(Feb. 2004): 153–62.

103. D'Inzeo, G., et al. "Microwave effects on acetylcholine-induced channels in cultured chick myotubes." *Bioelectromagnetics.* 9(4)(1988): 363–72.

104. Chiang, H., et al. "Health effects of environmental electromagnetic fields." *J. Bioelectricity.* 8(1989):127–31.

105. Kolodynski, A.A., and V.V. Kolodynska. "Motor and psychological functions of school children living in the area of the Skrunda Radio Location Station in Latvia." *Sci Total Environ.* 180(1)(1996): 87–93.

106. Firstenberg, A. "Electromagnetic Fields (EMF) Killing Fields." *The Ecologist.* 34(5)(June 1, 2004).

107. Santini, R., et al. "Investigation on the health of people living near mobile telephone relay stations: I/Incidence according to distance and sex." *Pathol Biol.* 50(6)(July 2002): 369–73.

108. Navarro, E.A., et al. "The microwave syndrome: a preliminary study in Spain." *Electromagnetic Biology and Medicine.* 22(2-3)(2003): 161–69.

109. Dalsegg, Aud. "Mobile phone radiation gives Gro Harlem Brundtland headaches." *Dagbladet.* March 9, 2002.

110. Von Pohl, Freiherr Gustav. *Earth Currents – as Pathogenic Agents for Illness and the Development of Cancer.* Feucht: Freich Verlag, 1983. (Out of print)

111. Bachler, K. *Earth Radiation.* Wordmasters, 1989.

112. Pfeffer, G., et al. "Comparison of custom and prefabricated orthoses in the initial treatment of proximal plantar fasciitis." *Foot Ankle Int.* 20(4)(1999): 214–21.

113. Caruso, W., and G. Leisman. "The clinical utility of force/displacement analysis of muscle testing in applied kinesiology." *Intern. J. Neuroscience.* 106(2001): 147–57.

114. "America's number 1 health problem: Why is there more stress today?" The American Stress Institute. http://www.stress.org/americas. htm?AIS=fhrzrhjb.

115. "Communications Workers Union health, safety and environment committee stress survey." The Labour Research Department for the CWU. May 2001: 3.

116. Holmes, T.H., and R.H. Rahe. "The Social Readjustment Rating Scale." *J Psychosom Res.* 11(2)(1967): 213–18.

117. 2 Corinthians 11:26–27. Phillips JB. *The New Testament in Modern English.* New York: Macmillan, 1960.

118. Romans 8:38–39. *New King James Version.* Thomas Nelson, 1982.

119. Brother Lawrence. *The practice of the presence of God.* Fleming H. Revel Company, 1958.

120. Keller, Helen. http://www.quotationspage.com/quotes/Helen_Keller.

121. Hershey, Jr., R. "Rise in death rate after new year is tied to the will to see 2000." *New York Times.* January 15, 2000.

122. Klemmer and Associates, Inc. 1340 Commerce St, Suite G, Petaluma, CA 94954. www.klemmer.com.

123. Ritchie, M.A. *Spirit of the rain forest: a yanomamo shaman's story.* Island Lake, IL: Island Lake Press, 2000.

124. Jones, P. "Chief Shoefoot's rebuke." *Touchstone.* Sept./Oct. 1998.

125. Daniel 10:13.

126. Luke 10:17.

127. Mark 13:34.

128. Matthew 17:21; Mark 9:29.

129. Sidney, S., et al. "Television viewing and cardiovascular risk factors in young adults: the CARDIA study." *Ann Epidemiol.* 6(2)(Mar. 1996): 154–59.

130. Piraro, Dan. *Bizarro*. King Features. June 2, 2006.

131. Brother Lawrence, op. cit. 14.

132. Ibid. 30-31.

133. 2 Corinthians 12:2-4.

134. 1 Corinthians 15:36; 42-44.

135. Acts 14:19.

136. Revelation 5:11.

137. Matthew 25:21.

Index

About the Author
Dale Peterson, M.D.

Dr. Peterson is a graduate of the University of Minnesota, College of Medicine. He completed a residency in Family Medicine at the University of Oklahoma. He also earned a Masters Degree in Biblical Studies from Pacific College of Graduate Studies.

Dr. Peterson practiced briefly in northern Wisconsin prior to serving as the assistant director of the Eau Claire Family Medicine residency program. In 1978 he moved to Edmond, Oklahoma, where he had a full-time family practice for over twenty years. He is a past Chief of Staff of the Edmond Hospital and a past president of the Oklahoma Academy of Family Physicians. He was active in teaching for many years as a Clinical Professor of Family Medicine through the Oklahoma University Health Sciences Center.

Dr. Peterson left his full-time family practice on March 1, 1999 to be able to consult with individuals who are seeking ways to restore and maintain their health through improved nutrition and other lifestyle changes. He founded the *Wellness Clubs of America* to give people access to credible information on supporting and maintaining their health. He created the *Center to Expose Iatrogenic Medicine* to alert physicians and patients alike of the dangers of medications and common medical procedures.

Dr. Peterson has an intense interest in the design of the human body and how, given proper nutrition and support, the body is able to halt the progression of disease and restore health. His monthly wellness letter, *Health By Design*, and his website, www.drdalepeterson.com, provide helpful information to individuals interested in preventing and conquering health challenges.

Dr. Peterson speaks regularly on subjects related to health and nutrition. He hosted a weekly radio program, *Your Health Matters*, on KTOK in Oklahoma City for five years. Since 2001, he has addressed questions from across the nation on the *Wellness Clubs of America* weekly teleconference. He has made numerous television appearances on the Trinity Broadcasting Network and he is currently a regular guest on radio programs across the country.

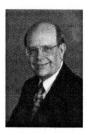

Contact Information

By Mail: Health by Design
1006 West Taft, #342
Sapulpa, OK 74066

By E-mail: info@drdalepeterson.com
Website: www.drdalepeterson.com